W9-BIH-037

Date: 1/3/20

618.928 LJU
Ljung, Ynge,
Finding your lost child :
understanding allergies,

Finding Your Lost Child

PALM BEACH COUNTY
LIBRARY SYSTEM
3650 SUMMIT BLVD.
WEST PALM BEACH, FL 33406

FINDING *Your Lost Child*

Understanding Allergies,
Nutrition, and Detox
in Autism, ADHD and
Children on the Spectrum

YNGE LJUNG

NEW YORK

LONDON • NASHVILLE • MELBOURNE • VANCOUVER

FINDING Your Lost Child

Understanding Allergies, Nutrition, and Detox in Autism, ADHD and Children on the Spectrum

© 2019 Ynge Ljung

All rights reserved. No portion of this book may be reproduced, stored in a retrieval system, or transmitted in any form or by any means—electronic, mechanical, photocopy, recording, scanning, or other—except for brief quotations in critical reviews or articles, without the prior written permission of the publisher.

Published in New York, New York, by Morgan James Publishing in partnership with Difference Press. Morgan James is a trademark of Morgan James, LLC. www. MorganJamesPublishing.com

The Morgan James Speakers Group can bring authors to your live event. For more information or to book an event visit The Morgan James Speakers Group at www.TheMorganJamesSpeakersGroup.com.

ISBN 9781642791440 paperback
ISBN 9781642791457 eBook
Library of Congress Control Number: 2018907232

Cover & Interior Design by:
Christopher Kirk
www.GFSstudio.com

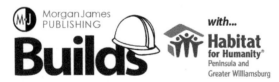

In an effort to support local communities, raise awareness and funds, Morgan James Publishing donates a percentage of all book sales for the life of each book to Habitat for Humanity Peninsula and Greater Williamsburg.

Get involved today! Visit
www.MorganJamesBuilds.com

To all the children and families in the world who are suffering from the pandemic of autism.

Table of Contents

Foreword

I have been simply amazed at the number of symptoms that can be directly related back to an allergy.

The medical profession states there are three symptoms that occur when an allergy is present: runny nose, watery eyes, and a rash. According to the medical profession, if you don't have one of these symptoms, you don't have an allergy.

It's been my experience as a natural health practitioner and a Higher Guidance Life Coach, that an allergic reaction can manifest in literally ANY abnormal symptom you can have: joint pain, fibromyalgia, mood disorders, metabolic issues, headaches, and even more astounding, autism, Tourette's, bi-polar, and anxiety.

Ynge's book brings a much-needed awareness of allergies and how they can be the root cause of health and mood disorders of the young and old alike.

My own awareness of the dramatic and unfortunate effect of unusual allergies began over 29 years ago when I was pregnant with my first son. As any good mom would do, I began taking prenatal vitamins. Unfortunately, I had severe diarrhea the entire first trimester. It was so severe and excruciating that I would find myself lying on the floor, cramping up from the pain.

A medical doctor did a complete check-up and said I was deficient in iron and consequently, anemic. He advised me to continue taking my prenatal vitamins. Other than that, he saw no explanation for my diarrhea.

Thirteen weeks into the pregnancy, a friend suggested my problems might be with my prenatal vitamins. The idea seemed crazy since I knew I needed the nutrients and wanted to resolve my anemia. Nonetheless, I stopped taking them and was astounded to experience a complete regulating of my bowel movements within a day.

I assumed the problem was that I had a bad brand so I bought a very expensive one at the health food store. After just one capsule, the diarrhea came back. I experimented with three other brands, all with the same immediate effect. Fourteen weeks into my pregnancy, I stopped all prenatal vitamins and miraculously had no more issues.

Even so, after that many weeks of severe diarrhea, I had lost significant electrolytes. I believe it was the reason I had a very difficult birth, which ended in a Caesarean section.

When I was pregnant with my second child, I stayed away from prenatal vitamins and instead worked with herbs to keep my iron count up. Even when pregnant with my third child, I still kept away from prenatal vitamins but didn't understand what was going on.

Prior to my fourth pregnancy, I came across a book called *Say Good-Bye-BYE to Illness* by Devi S. Nambudripad. The book explains that there are many unusual allergies and even components of foods that never present in the typical ways: runny nose, watery eyes, and a rash.

That's when the light bulb turned on, and I instantly understood I was allergic to iron! Prenatal vitamins are high in iron, which caused severe diarrhea for me. Now, knowing what I know about unusual allergies, I can look back at my pregnancy and clearly see that I was anemic because I was allergic to the iron in the prenatal vitamins. Weirdly, iron was the very thing I needed yet my body rejected it.

I believe in what Ynge shares in this book and the dramatic healing that can take place with The Allergy Kit. I believe it because I lived it. The Allergy Kit is a brilliant technique, that Ynge created, allowing you to treat yourself and your family in your own home

I cleared my iron allergy and was able to take prenatal vitamins without incident during my fourth pregnancy. It was an easy, natural birth. I continued to work on all four of my children using The Allergy Kit throughout their lives.

I know firsthand how frustrating it can be to uncover the mystery behind an ailment. Ynge will give you many possibilities to explore as you go on your journey. Awareness is everything!

Jean Slatter,
author of *Hiring the Heavens* and
founder of The Higher Guidance Life Coach Program.

Autism Spectrum Disorders and Allergies

"The gut is the source of all illnesses."

– Hippocrates

Early in my career, I began to see a few new types of patients – some of them had been diagnosed with autism or on the autism spectrum disorders (ASD), others not yet diagnosed. But with time, I saw more and more kids with these kinds of problems. My concern for my patients led me to begin researching autism from a holistic perspective.

During two decades of research, I gained deeper insights into autism, allergies, nutrition, and detoxification. I created this book to bring this information together in one place to enable you to achieve better health for your entire family.

From a holistic nutritional perspective and according to Hippocrates, "All illness begins in the gut." More and more holistic doctors are starting to understand the truth in this, and scientists are working on the "new thing" – the microbiome.

Children with ADD, ADHD, autism, Asperger's, or any other form of ASD, all have allergies. Some of these children suffer from very severe allergies as the result of a compromised digestive system.

The gut is not called the second brain for nothing – it controls all the functions in the body and also the brain!

Dietary changes can improve the health of anyone suffering from a condition such as autism, since they all have compromised digestive systems and multiple food and environmental allergies. In some cases, eliminating allergens from their diets can result in rapid improvement in healing the gut and a lot of the typical ASD symptoms.

Most children coping with ASD also have other health problems besides their allergies. This group may experience subtler enhancement in overall health after subtracting allergens from their diets. However, patients of all ages, and at every point on the ASD, can benefit from the allergen elimination approach, together with lifestyle changes.

Healing the digestive tract by eliminating identified allergens, and changing the diet can improve the overall health and well-being of all ASD children.

The allergy elimination approach clears up their digestive problems such as diarrhea/constipation, irritable bowel syndrome (IBS), or leaky gut, for example– problems which the mainstream medical establishment tends to view as coincidental rather than correlated to ASD. As a result of eliminating allergic reactions, children with an ASD or on the autism spectrum become less prone to tantrums and their interactions with others becomes easier.

Why I Created The Allergy Kit

I started to experiment with different combinations and treatment protocols and had very good results!

But, there were many kids I couldn't reach – living too far away from a practitioner or the cost was too much. I wanted to be able to help them too, and that is how The Allergy Kit was born! I worked in my office with my new technique for years, before I finally was ready to present it to the public!

The year was 2006.

Since then I have reached thousands of families!

This book is written for you who feel hopeless, because your doctors say there is no solution. You are exhausted, your family is falling apart, and you don't know how to manage or raise your child. Worst of all, you are seeing your child suffering and you don't know how to help.

Following the advice in this book and working with a functional doctor, you could find your lost child again! I have seen the possible changes that can happen!

This is what I want to show you:

Where to start

- What foods to eliminate for starters
- Cleaning out the pantry
- How to read labels

Different diets:

- SFCF – Gluten-Free, Casein-Free Diet
- SCD – Specific Carbohydrate Diet™

- BED – Body Ecology Diet
- Nourishing Traditions Weston A. Price Diet
- Other diets
- Nutrition

Lifestyle

- Cleaning out the house from chemicals:
    - Cleaning products
    - Detergents and fabric softeners
    - Shampoos and soaps
    - Air fresheners

Detoxing from Toxins

Autism Spectrum Disorders (ASD) and Allergies

With the autism spectrum disorders (ASD) being a pandemic, we will have to change the opinion that schools, universities, and the general population have of what is "different" and what is "normal" and teach about acceptance and love for each other.

It may take time, it may not! One child in four today may become autistic or be on the spectrum. We just have to get used to it and work harder on changing the vaccine schedule, making it a choice to start to vaccinate at a later age when the brain barrier is developed and the risk becomes much lower. Or make it a choice, period. Let the parents decide!

There may be genetic factors causing autism, but if researchers are looking at genes, they're looking in the wrong place.

Even if the causes are or were due to the genes, the environmental factors are so much greater! These disorders are neurological, like for example Alzheimer's or Parkinson's and even schizophrenia, and they can all be improved with a different diet and detox!

Children have a heavy vaccination schedule from the very first day of life, when they get a shot for hepatitis B.

The baby's brain barrier is not developed until they are around three years old, so the neurotoxins from the vaccinations go straight to their brain!

At that point, it is impossible to know if there is any damage done. However, following the current vaccine schedule, some children may react more with each vaccine, but not enough for alarm, so the parents are told it is normal for the babies to have a reaction.

And then, one day, life has changed!

You had a happy, smart, beautiful baby, and all of a sudden, they are not developing as they should.

They often have diarrhea and sometimes constipation, and their digestion problems just get worse and worse, and you don't know what to do.

Tummy pain is a constant. Why?

Maybe it starts out as a neurological problem, but now it is a whole-body disorder!

Every single child on the autism spectrum has food allergies, and other allergies too, but since we build up our immune system through absorbing the food, having food allergies makes it impossible to regulate the digestion, and autoimmune disorders may develop, adding to all the other problems.

Whatever some doctors say - at least pediatricians who give the vaccinations and telling the parents they are safe - **the root of ASD comes from the vaccinations** and that they are given at such an early age, that the brain barrier is not yet developed.

This is probably the third generation of vaccinated people having kids, with every generation getting weaker and weaker, so what can we expect?

These children are very sensitive and not only are they being vaccinated at a very young age, they are also exposed to all the toxins in the environment.

Babies born today have close to 300 different toxins and chemicals in their umbilical cord, transferred from their mothers. Also, not only is the air filled with exhaust from cars and airplanes, factories spew out their chemicals and toxins and all food is sprayed with herbicides and pesticides, which we then eat. And the list goes on!

Unfortunately, kids with ASD can't detox heavy metals and other chemicals. Eating food they are allergic to, and being toxic at the same time, makes life very difficult for these kids. They are in pain! They can't sleep, they feel horrible when they eat food they can't tolerate– it's a mess.

These children have all kinds of problems:

- Leaky gut
- SIBO
- Candida

- Colitis
- Diarrhea/constipation
- Any kind of digestive problem

Food allergies to:

- Salicylates
- Oxalates
- Amines
- Electromagnetic frequencies
- And more

Mineral deficiencies and imbalances are common. Different foods can have different reactions. Salicylate containing food can create psychological and behavioral symptoms.

Wheat can make these children spacey, even giving rise to seizures. Sometimes the seizures are so faint that for a little bit of time, the child just stares out in the air and seems unconscious of the environment and doesn't respond to their name when called.

Electromagnetic Fields and Electromagnetic Radio Waves (EMF/EMR) can give rise to insomnia and many things you wouldn't even relate to the culprits, since you can't see frequencies.

Is this the cause for some kid's super sensitivity to noise and touch?

There are still so many things we don't know, and new things are being researched all the time, but there are some basics: food and toxins – the microbiome and the gut!

Those are the first things that need to be taken care of, and also what will give the best results fastest!

Where to Start

Allergies and What You Need to Know

Holistic health experts use a more comprehensive approach to the concept of allergies than allopathic (traditional western medicine) doctors. The allopathic approach only identifies as allergens those substances that cause people to sneeze, break out in hives, or experience other readily identifiable symptoms, mostly through testing.

The holistic health understanding of allergies on the other hand, observes that our environments may be filled with substances that trigger subtle allergic reactions in many people. These allergic reactions cause a gradual loss of digestive system efficiency. These flaws in the digestive system (which often are not diagnosed as a health problem at all or only diagnosed after years of suffering) create a ripple effect of decreased health throughout the body, mainly by depleting the immune system.

In recent years, the importance of our bacteria and other "critters" living in our bodies, called the microbiome, has been shown to be much more important than earlier believed. Our own cells comprise of 10 percent of all the cells in the body; the other 90 percent is bacteria, viruses, fungi, and pathogens! This means we're just the host. That also means we have to keep the balance of microbiomes in check in order to stay healthy and happy!

With the arrival of GMOs in the 1990's and the immense use of herbicide and pesticide, our gut-health has ever since been compromised, and we are out of balance.

More on GMOs in a later chapter.

The Link Between Allergies and ASD

Children with ASD are extremely sensitive. We don't know exactly why. It could be from inheriting the parents' immune system, it could be from being damaged by the heavy metals in the vaccines, and it could also be due to eating non-organic, toxic food. It is most probably from a combination of all these things.

We make our immune system from the digestive system. If we can't absorb the food for one reason or another, for example because of allergies, the immune system weakens, which affects the total health of the body.

Then the next thing that happens is that the body gets nutrient deficient. Adding supplements doesn't help since the body is also allergic or sensitive to these nutrients and builds up "toxins" from the supplements that should be good for them.

With the rejection comes a reaction, which is the so-called allergic reaction. Often the reaction is not understood as that since it is outside "normal" allergic reactions.

Temper tantrums, for example, can be an allergic reaction to dairy and/or wheat. Not understanding that the tantrums are an allergic reaction, parents often get criticized for bad parenting when they take their kids out for pizza. Has that ever happened to you?

Head banging and seizures are also allergic reactions, as well as the child not having eye contact.

This is why allergies play such an important role in treating ASD.

Everybody may not have allergies, but every single child and person on the spectrum does! They often have many allergies, not only to foods, but they can also be to dogs, cats, smells, noise, lights, fabrics, and so on. They can be allergic to absolutely everything, even to parents and siblings! Allergies most usually start with food allergies. Your baby may also be reacting to your milk, depending on what you're eating!

Treating your child for allergies is the first step and may be the most important step in seeing an improved difference in your child. In addition, changing the diets for what is best for your child, and also looking at and changing lifestyle, can be life changing for your whole family!

The following is part of Christine's story, a mother of three:

When I started the kit, the very first thing I noticed was with my son. It was amazing, after the very first vial, after 48 hours, he was a completely different child. We had moved from up north to Colorado, and two years later we noticed that his nose was running and didn't make the connection to food allergies. We thought it was environmental, so we didn't realize the severe egg allergy he had. For the last nine months, we could never get him, to sit down at the dinner table with us. We had tried everything; it didn't matter what we did or didn't do, he would not sit down with us and we really thought it was a behavior issue. He was very aggressive with his sister, very short-tempered with her. He hadn't played with her for the last nine months, and that was gone in 48 hours after starting the kit!

Once you see the difference, you will become passionate about healing your child and maybe helping other mothers, too!

Allergies – Where Do They Come From?

The immune system starts in the gut. You can be born with allergies, maybe inherited them from parents or other relatives.

It could also be the other way around. Due to the food being toxic – not grown in rich soil and/or not picked fresh, or the child's diet contains too much sugar and sugary foods, processed foods and fast foods – the gut gets sick and affected. This often results in allergies, IBS, Crohn's or leaky gut, just to mention a few.

With a leaky gut, food particles leak out into the bloodstream, which then leads to allergies and intolerances.

I also believe now that the last several generations have been vaccinated, everybody's immune system is getting weaker and so our bodies today are more toxic. The babies are born weaker and more sensitive, and their digestive systems don't work optimally. If our bodies could absorb all the nutrients from the good food we eat, we would never get sick because our immune system would be strong and supportive.

This is not the case anymore and that's why I started to work with allergies. I could see the connection everywhere: headaches, migraines, sciatica, shoulder, hip problems, and so on.

With children, it is very obvious that something is not right. They get an ear infection and are then given antibiotics. After a little while, they have a strep throat and they get antibiotics again. The problem is that we don't associate the idea of the child's food allergies and infections or inflammations together with their allergic reactions.

Instead of eliminating the foods or the allergy, we treat the symptoms with antibiotics, not the cause – allergies. We're looking in the wrong place! If a child doesn't want to drink their milk, there is a reason! They probably don't feel well having dairy and that's why they refuse it. The same thing happens with other foods, too.

To add further insult to injury, the antibiotics destroy the digestive system, the GI tract, enzymes, and bacteria, both good and bad. Some people suffer from this side effect all their lives, not knowing what hit them! If your child suffers from diarrhea, for example, it could be from having an ear infection and taking antibiotics for it!

I had a patient – a little girl only two years old – who was brought to me by her father. She was very small for her age and wasn't thriving. She got sick almost twice a month with ear infections or strep throat, and this had been going on for a while. The father was very worried and felt so bad that he couldn't do anything for his darling daughter.

I treated her for a milk allergy at the first visit and after that she never had an ear infection again!

Then we had to work on her diet and treat the candida she had developed from all the antibiotics she had been given. Soon she started to thrive and grow and turned into a happy little girl! Her father was very happy, too!

The Second Brain

It is a well-known fact that the gut is considered the second brain! The gut can affect absolutely everything in the body! The vagus nerve goes all the way from the brain through the neck, lungs, and the other organs down to the gut.

For example, remember when you had too much to eat after a Thanksgiving meal? Everybody is totally out of it – can't think and can hardly move. That's how it feels.

ASD kids are very toxic and have difficulties detoxing, much more difficult than for other folks.

A lot of the toxins are in the brain as heavy metals, mostly from vaccinations. These metals also affect the digestion. The combination of antibiotics killing good and bad bacteria, leading to candida, together with heavy metals is very damaging to the brain.

Taking into consideration that practically every child has had several rounds of antibiotics, the gut is overgrown with fungus, or candida, and together with the heavy metal toxicity, this situation becomes a **whole-body disorder**, not only a neurological disorder! The environment, as well as what they eat and drink, greatly affects their situation.

As a whole-body disorder, treating with proper food and detox, the child can greatly improve in every aspect of their life!

The Allergy Kit

In this chapter, I'm going to show you the first steps you need to take to get yourself on the right path for helping your child. Then we'll get into the different diets and nutrition; however, the success of the diets works best when coupled with The Allergy Kit.

The Allergy Kit helps treat the symptoms of the allergic reactions and helps to eliminate the allergen. The Allergy Kit is energy medicine. You don't take anything, nor do you put anything on your skin.

By treating with The Allergy Kit, it will help to eliminate some of the negative reactions from foods and other substances, and thus accelerate the efficacy of other, adjunct treatments for sensitive and compromised gut issues. Cravings are eliminated as well as many typical ASD symptoms, like stimming, avoidance of eye contact, temper tantrums, and more.

Improvement may not happen immediately since every child is unique, and each child will respond in different ways. It is recommended to do the treatment at night since it is very relaxing and makes them sleep well.

You also have to remember that there are several different treatments that work together synergistically, and you can't do only one thing for a couple of days and think this is it, and then get disappointed if it doesn't work!

The Allergy Kit works together with the diet and with the detox, so don't stop any of these, or any other treatments you're doing.

The first treatment is for milk, chicken, eggs, and vitamin C.

Eric was very aggressive with his sisters. He couldn't sit still, and he would never sit down at the table with the rest of the family for dinner, which irritated his father immensely. After this very first treatment, Eric calmed down and was like a different child! It changed the whole family.

The mother was elated when she told me the story, and the relationship with her husband totally changed to the better! She had been very worried that he was thinking about leaving her, which happens so often in families with these issues!

The second treatment is for sugars and vitamin B.

This treatment is immensely important for many reasons.

It destroys the sugar balance, and consuming sugars, whether it is in its raw form or from sugary foods, like bread, pasta, pizza, ketchup, fruit juices, and sodas, is the way to obesity and diabetes.

Beet sugar is a BT ready and a genetically modified organism (GMO food). That it is BT ready means it is a pesticide (and classified as that), not a food!

Wherever sugars are added, so are high fructose corn syrup (HFCS) and corn syrup, which are also GMO foods.

Have you noticed how super excited and hyper the kids get when they eat sweets?

Once I took my grandkids to Cold Stone for ice cream. After just two teaspoons of ice cream, the younger five-year-old, started to run up and down the place, which was long and narrow, and didn't have time to finish his treat! Guess what I didn't do any more?

The third treatment is for toxins.

We are all toxic! Babies today are born with close to 300 different toxins and chemicals in their umbilical cord!

Unfortunately, ASD children have great difficulty in detoxing and often feel horrible and don't know why, unable to express their feelings either. Often these feelings come out as anger and outbursts, sometimes as temper tantrums. It is not their fault!

Six-year-old Andrew stopped hitting his siblings and peers after having gone through the toxin treatment.

The fourth treatment is for vaccinations. *Check the Chapter 5 for more info about vaccinations and vaccines.*

Most ASD children have been vaccinated, or their mother has had some of the recommended shots. The vaccines also add to the toxic load through the heavy metals in the vaccines. The treatments for vaccines and toxins are very important, and sometimes the change in the child can be great! The heavy metals in the shots are stored in the brain, and they are neurotoxins. They are very difficult to get rid of, but so important to do so!

I had one client, Hannah, who was diagnosed as ADHD. She had a lot of problems due to her anger. She was adopted and knew it. She hated her mother and fought with her all the time about everything. She loved her father, though. She also had big problems in school.

One of her classmates, Claudia, was, according to Hannah, always fighting with her, and sometimes they had fistfights. They seemed to hate each other and their fights and screaming were a constant disturbance – just like at home, where Hannah fought with her mom!

After I did Hannah's fourth treatment, the one for vaccinations, her behavior improved 180 degrees! When I asked her on her follow-up visit how everything was, she said her mother had changed and Claudia didn't fight with her anymore! It certainly was amazing!

I can't remember a single child, who hasn't had some kind of positive change after the vaccination treatment with The Allergy Kit!

The fifth treatment is for sugars again, plus candida.

This is a sugar treatment again because of the importance of being able to stay away from sugar, and thus treat candida. Candida is a malady that practically all ASD children suffer from and is the reason why they crave sweets and processed and fast foods. Please refer to *The Body Ecology Diet in* Chapter 3 for more information on candida.

It is very important to read labels – there is sugar in almost everything! As I mentioned above in the second treatment, sugar is dangerous!

One of my patients brought in her 15-year-old daughter, Cherie, who was so tired and depressed, had fuzzy thinking, and couldn't remember anything. This was so bad that she couldn't even go to school.

They had been to four different doctors who couldn't find anything wrong with her, and one of them wanted to put her on drugs for depression.

When I saw her and checked her tongue, it was completely covered with a thick, white coat (a typical indication of candida). I put her on the BET diet and gave her some herbs.

The change happened within a week. She felt like a totally different person, could think again, went back to school, and her mom didn't have to worry that something was dreadfully wrong with her. Knowing now what set the symptoms in motion, they know they can control their diets!

The sixth treatment is for grains and corn.

This is also something these children will crave, often for cereals laced with sugars and food colors. Some get evident reactions from this like belly pain, rash, etc., but most do not. The reactions could be in the form of headache or being tired.

I had another little patient, Jon, 4 years old, who always had an upset stomach – either he had diarrhea, or he was constipated, and always seemed to be in pain. He didn't play with his siblings. Often, he would sit and not pay attention to anything, just stare out in the air. His mom used to give him either sugar-coated cereals, or pancakes made with wheat flour for breakfast. He loved both of these foods and used to ask for them every day.

After working with him on grains, he had a big change! His stools normalized, he started to talk more, and play with his siblings. He was a much more harmonious person and so was the whole family!

These are the first basic treatments. Many other treatments follow these.

Some kids have already been tested for allergies, so the parents know what they are allergic to. Others haven't been tested and the parents may not even know their children have allergies at all!

The autistic children all have to be treated for these first allergens before any other treatments for allergies are done. It helps them to strengthen their immune system and also to become aware of other allergies they have.

To eliminate these basic allergies will help with any of the other special diets. It will help them with their cravings. Different foods have different kinds of reactions. Eggs or chicken can be the cause of lack of eye contact, for example. Milk or other dairy products can make them spacey, aggressive, stimming, and irritable among other things. Sugars, high fructose corn syrup (HFCS), and other sweeteners can make them hyperactive and maybe aggressive.

They can be allergic to their clothes, carpets, the smell of a new car, their mattress, or things in the school, like crayons, paints on the walls – anything! Some are allergic to chemicals in the food, or to certain smells. They can be allergic to histamine in certain foods. They can even be allergic to themselves or someone in the family – parents or siblings – showing up in how they get along with other people or not.

There are a lot of other allergens we often don't put together with different reactions. For example, cotton today is a GMO product and sprayed with a lot of glyphosate. When you buy cotton, you think you're using the best for your child, but is it the best if he is sensitive to toxins?

People who crave certain foods are often allergic to that specific food. Maybe this is because the body needs that nutrient but can't absorb it, or maybe it does something to their head that they like on a subconscious level.

These cravings make it more difficult to have the children stop these foods. They may become very angry, and often the parents give up and let the children have what they want. But this is not in the child's best interest! Remember, you are the parent!

It will take willpower and maybe fights, but it is important for parents/caregivers to stand their ground!

Using The Allergy Kit will greatly help since it takes away the cravings once that specific allergy is cleared!

It can be hard work putting the puzzle pieces together – but it is worth it, so don't give up.

To help your child maintain success the first thing to do is to pay attention to the pantry.

Cleaning Up the Pantry

One essential thing to do is go through your pantry and throw away (or give away) everything that contains sugar, HFCS, anything with artificial sweeteners first, together with everything that contains wheat and/or gluten. Sorry, but the pasta has to go, too!

This is not fun ,but it has to be done.

All preservatives and pickles have to go the same way! I hope you don't have too much of these things or it may feel as if you're throwing away a fortune, and you probably are! But the goal is to get your child to feel good! It may not feel so good for *you* when he asks for something that is in the trash, but it can't be helped. This has to be done!

You have to let go of everything with food coloring, with monosodium glutamate (MSG) or anything with the other names for it, mentioned above.

You will have to be brave! Maybe the other members of the family will complain too, but they also have to let it go. After a while, you will all feel better and not miss the old foods too much.

It's like an old friend that leaves. In the beginning there is a big hole, but with time the hole heals, and you forget, and maybe even realize it was good to part from them.

I know that this is one of the most difficult things to do and this is almost the first thing in changing your lifestyle. Until you have finished this stage, you can't move forward to the next steps, which are avoiding some foods to eliminate the allergies.

It's quite easy to learn about the clean eating lifestyle, but following it can be difficult and a major shock (a good one) to your body. One of the main foundations of clean eating is cutting out and avoiding processed foods. This is very important, and I can't repeat it enough when you have an ASD child. Doing so will prevent the consumption of unhealthy, and sometimes very harmful, additives.

Processed foods are hard on your body and have been connected to serious health complications, including cardiovascular disease and obesity. They can contain so many bad ingredients that are difficult on your liver and for you to digest, and those harmful ingredients and additives are often then stored in the body.

The whole family will benefit from this change in lifestyle!

Reading the ingredient list and nutritional information on the side of pre-made, packaged, and processed foods can be a real wake-up call if you haven't read it before. Processed foods can have an alarming amount of sodium, fat, and sugar. To make it worse, the serving size is often only half or less of what you'd regularly eat. Next time you're shopping, skip processed foods to eat clean in order to greatly improve your and your family's health.

This is a list that pinpoints the most pesticide-prone produce in America. Based on data collected by the U.S. Department of Agriculture and Food and Drug Administration (USDA), it is meant to help us make better-informed shopping choices – not to stop eating our veggies! This list will help you to know when you must buy organic and when you can get away with buying non-organic. Try to buy local and organic, preferably not packed!

Foods to avoid for starters

One of the biggest problems the ASD kids have is that they can't detox like other people. They are often constipated, making them even more toxic, with tummy aches and headaches adding to injury. Foods to avoid may be a difficult step to take initially, especially if the whole family is used to eating the so-called American diet, with a lot of processed, sugary foods. This is when you have to be strong in order to see the results you wish to see!

To eliminate ASD kids' allergies is of the greatest importance. They have to avoid certain foods as well, for starters milk/dairy, sugars and wheat.

Caseomorphins and gluteomorphins, the food opioids are morphine-like substances formed during digestion of casein in cow's milk and in wheat respectively. The protein in cow's milk; casein, makes up 80 – 90 percent of the total protein content, while goat's milk only contains up to 2 percent. This protein causes damage to the intestinal lining in the colon and is the reason why they have to stay away from these products even after being desensitized for milk and wheat, at least until their gut is repaired and digestion is under control. An alternative is to maybe try goat's milk.

Casein

Casein from dairy turns into caseomorphine, and gluten from wheat turns into gliadin morphine. When consuming dairy or wheat, some people behave as if they were drunk, others can't think clearly. Some kids start banging their head – they're trying to release something and of course parents don't understand why the kids are behaving in such ways. How could you?

Wheat

Wheat has been hybridized since the 1930s, and during this time, 18 proteins that didn't exist before, developed in the gluten. One of them is gliadin. That's the one that turns into an opiate and affects certain people in a negative way, and also makes them very addicted to it. I have patients who, when I say to them that the wheat has to go, throw their hands in the air and say: *No, no! You can't take away my bread!* That is because of the addiction!

Why are there so many more negative reactions today than before?

Apart from this extra protein in gluten, in the past, the bread was prepared differently. The dough would be prepared the night before baking the bread, so the gluten was more consumed through the fermentation period that took place for several hours. Today the bread is made, from beginning to the end, in two hours!

Another thing that happens today is that a couple of days before harvest, the wheat is sprayed with Roundup, which contains the toxic chemical glyphosate, which makes the toxins go straight up to the grains that we consume!

How come the so-called gluten intolerance has risen hundreds of percent the last 20 years? Is it really gluten intolerance or is it toxin intolerance?

I, myself, used to have pain in my hips to a point that I couldn't sleep on my sides for several years. On top of that, sometimes I got a horrible pain in either hip, so bad I could hardly walk and had to hold onto walls or whatever was close. One day I had bread in a restaurant and after the meal I could hardly get up from the table! I realized then, that I had a reaction to the wheat. I did treat myself for wheat, but it didn't work for non-organic wheat. I then stopped eating any kind of wheat. It has been several years, and I have no more hip pain! I can eat anything with gluten – just not wheat!

I can eat every kind of bread they have in Israel, and I can eat most bread in Europe (they import some wheat from America). So, I know I am not gluten intolerant, I am American-wheat intolerant, and I don't think I am the only one. It is probably the toxins from the glyphosate.

Sugars

Sugars are the worst epidemic in the western world. One hundred years ago, sugars and sweets were very uncommon because only the rich could afford them. The consumption of sweets has now gone up to 100 pounds per person per year! Now, sugar beets and corn, from which sugars are made, are GMO foods and highly toxic!

Most of the sweeteners are in soft drinks that people drink instead of water, and thus, totally undermining their health, making obesity and diabetes the leading health issues in this country, with all the other diseases following as a result. Consuming all these sweet drinks depletes the body of micronutrients, producing hunger, obesity and nutrient deficiency.

Sweetener #1: High Fructose Corn Syrup

High Fructose Corn Syrup, or HFCS is in almost all processed or fast food. The average American consumes 63 pounds of HFCS a year!

- HFCS is a GMO food.
- It depletes chromium, magnesium, zinc and copper from the body. (The zinc/copper in ASD is very often out of balance).

- It does not trigger leptin (the feel full hormone), causing overeating.
- It causes insulin to spike, which in the not so long run, can lead to diabetes.
- Twenty percent of all the calories children consume come from HFCS

Sweetener #2: Sugar

Sugar, if it is not organic, is a genetically modified organism.

One thing for certain we know about GMO is that it is heavily sprayed with Roundup, containing Glyphosate, which is very damaging to the gut.

If your child has had antibiotics in their life, they probably also suffer from candida, or yeast overgrowth in the intestines.

Candida has many symptoms, like gas, bloating, constipation/diarrhea, itchiness in the groin or armpit, chronic stuffy nose, restlessness, hyperactivity or being very tired, behaving as if drunk or on drugs, and a constant craving for sugar. The sugar is necessary for the candida bacteria to be able to reproduce and that's why they crave it so much. It is like an addiction and often very difficult to take away.

Treating for sugar allergy with The Allergy Kit makes it easier for them to get rid of the cravings.

Sweetener #3: Artificial Sweeteners

Artificial sweeteners are all detrimental to anyone's health, but to kids with ASD it is poison. Eliminate all artificial sweeteners: NutraSweet, Equal, aspartame, Sweet-n-low, saccharin, Truvia, and anything that is not pure stevia. Other sugars affect the neurons in the brain in a bad way and can cause headaches, migraine, and also seizures and hyperactivity.

Warning: Artificial sweeteners cut the good gut bacteria in half with each consumption!

The results of avoiding/eliminating these culprits will be amazing and you will be very happy going through with these changes!

Soda

Soda is probably the worst drink in the world! There is not one single item in the ingredient list that has any nutritional value whatsoever! Its first ingredient is high fructose corn syrup, followed by sugar. One soda contains 12 spoons of sugar!

Do you think anyone could possibly consume that in the crude form, one spoon after the other? I don't think so.

In addition to the sweeteners, soda contains caramel color and other food colors, (some carcinogenic!), and these definitely cause hyperactivity in children! The list goes on. What about phosphoric acid, artificial flavors (MSG), sodium benzoate, brominated vegetable oil, calcium disodium, and more?

They all leach out important micronutrients, and the lack of them leads to many different disorders. A known fact is that in ASD kids there is an imbalance between zinc and copper, for example.

Most sodas have a pH value of 2! You can clean your car's chromium wheels with it, with very good result! Think what that can do to the teeth! As well as our gut!

Veggies and berries to avoid due to high toxicity:

- Strawberries (tops the list, having over 20 different pesticides)
- Spinach (comes next)
- Nectarines
- Apples
- Peaches
- Pears
- Cherries
- Grapes
- Celery
- Tomatoes
- Sweet bell peppers
- Potatoes

So, stay away from produce on this list, or buy them organic! How about growing your own organic vegetables. The tower garden makes it super easy. No soil, and very little space required!

Some clean food you can get non-organic

- Sweet corn (even though I don't recommend corn for ASD diets)
- Avocados (excellent food)

- Cabbage
- Onions
- Frozen sweet peas
- Asparagus
- Mangoes
- Eggplant (this is in the nightshade family, often allergies attributed to them)
- Kiwi
- Cauliflower
- Grapefruit

The clean eating trend is growing as people realize the benefits of changing not just their diet, but also their lifestyle to cut out processed foods and buy foods directly from the source.

When you start eating "clean", and your child sees you're all eating the same way, they will want to eat that way, too. Also, fresh, organic food tastes so much better.

Clean eating changes the way they eat, how much they eat, and when they eat. It encourages altering their diet so that they eat fresh produce and allowed grains, that are packed full of nutrients, as well as other foods that contain good fats to improve overall health. This lifestyle has many health benefits, including reducing the risk of cardiovascular disease, many types of cancers, and other medical problems, so it will be good for the whole family!

Being aware of the journey the food takes to make it to the plate cuts out additives, fillers, and other unnecessary products. Follow these clean eating points to reap the benefits of a trend that's sure to stay.

If you have a chance to grow your own food and to get your child involved, it can make a huge difference! If they grow their own food, they will want to eat it!

No processed foods

To avoid processed food is extremely important for your autistic child, and can avoid many unpleasant symptoms, like diarrhea, no eye contact, temper tantrums, and even seizures

– and, of course this is great for the whole family!

Avoid all processed foods. They contain all kinds of artificial flavors and colors, toxins, and chemicals. They are almost always served together with wheat in some form. They contain bleach and who knows what more.

To make sure you're buying the right types of food for your child, it's really important you learn to read the labels.

Learn How to Read Labels

This is not an easy task! We often don't even know what we're looking for! We see the package, it looks beautiful! The artistic rendering is very attractive, and it even says "natural!" What more do you want?

This packaging is very deceptive! Anything can be natural, but does that mean it is safe to consume? No – not at all! In many cases the design is designed to deceive you with a promise on the front of the package that this is a great, wholesome food and you forget to check the label on the side or backside, where you can see for yourself whether it is good or not.

You have to learn to read the labels! I can't repeat this enough!

This is extremely important if you want to help your child – and the whole family too, for that matter! When you start on this journey, you will be amazed at how much better everybody will feel, and you are going to want to learn more.

Learn how to identify foods that really are good for you and your child and learn how to stay away from foods that sound and look healthy but are deceiving you with great marketing ploys.

The front of the package is the marketing plan. The so-called "Nutrition Facts" are on the label. The most important, but often forgotten is the "Ingredient List". This is where you really get to know the product and what is in it, but most people don't think about reading this part.

To enhance the taste of foods, they add sugars, often in the form of HFCS and color, so it looks more appetizing! This is not mentioned on the front of the package! Only that it is a low-fat food and you can eat as much as you want!

You must to go to the "Ingredient List" to get the truth! You can see how much sugar, GMO corn oil, or soy, also a GMO food, has been added.

MSG is one of the worst food additives there is, especially for your child, because it is a neurotoxin.

Nowadays MSG has many misleading names to make sure you think it is something good!

Here are some hidden names of MSG in substances containing the highest percentage of factory created free glutamate, with MSG containing 78 percent:

- MSG gelatin calcium caseinate
- Monosodium glutamate hydrolyzed vegetable protein (HVP) textured protein
- Monopotassium glutamate hydrolyzed plant protein (HPP) yeast extract
- Glutamate autolyzed plant protein yeast food or nutrient
- Glutamic acid sodium caseinate autolyzed yeast

Reading labels is not easy, and information changes all the time. It is not easy to know what to believe or do.

But remember, the less ingredients, the better. Compare different brands; it can be very enlightening! Once you start reading labels, you will find out things you had never thought of and it can become an interesting journey.

Food manufacturers deliberately mislead consumers through false labeling. Products marked "gluten-free" on the package may not really mean gluten-free. Many times, manufacturers merely replace wheat with another grain containing gluten.

Also avoid any food whose ingredients contain numbers – numbers mean food coloring, which should be strictly avoided.

Avoid artificial sweeteners, including Splenda, as well as the so-called natural ones like Truvia, Malta, agave, sugars, yeast, added flavors and whey.

Fruits and vegetables are very important for healing. Lightly steaming vegetables makes them easier to digest, particularly for a sensitive leaky gut.

I suggest whole fruits rather than fruit juice for children with autism. Fruit juices cause high levels of sugar to enter the bloodstream, disrupting the blood sugar levels, affecting the whole endocrine system.

If they have candida, which they mostly do, cut down on fruits, too, especially apples and grapes.

Many parents give children fruit as a dessert after meals. While this may seem like a healthy alternative to sugary desserts, the timing of this style of eating inhibits digestion. It is best to eat fruits about 30 minutes before meals.

Most fruits move through the digestive system very quickly, in about fifteen minutes. Fruits eaten after a meal sit on top of the other food that takes longer to digest. As a result, the fruit ferments in the body rather than being digested.

In effect, by giving your child a fruit dessert, you are making wine in their stomach.

To make sure you have the right foods it's important to know where to shop.

Where and How to Shop

It is not easy to know how to shop and where to find the "right" stuff.

There is a book by Jayson Calton, PhD and his wife Mira Calton, CN, with the title *Rich Food, Poor Food.*

It's an excellent book, teaching you "the ultimate grocery purchasing system", a GPS in shopping smart and healthy while saving time and money!

They teach you where to go in the grocery store, whether it's Publix, Whole Foods, Trader Joe's, or any other store! You will learn where the dangers in foods and packages are lurking and how to look at the packages to know what the truth is! I strongly recommend it.

If you don't get the book, know that where you pick up your groceries is all around the store. With that I mean the four walls and what is on them: dairy and nondairy, fish and meat, and then vegetables

In the dairy aisle, stay away from all yogurts that are fat-free (processed) or contain berries (loaded with sugars). Choose organic and non-homogenized, if possible. The best is of course raw, unprocessed organic dairy!

Choose foods that contain live or active cultures, though I believe they die pretty quickly after the pasteurizing - they can't live there!

If you eat cheese, buy the imported cheeses - they don't have GMO's in Europe!

Eggs have to be organic! Pasture raised hens' eggs have seven times more beta carotene, three times more vitamin E, two times more omega-3s, and two-thirds more vitamin A!

Standard factory eggs are produced by abused hens living under no acceptable circumstances, fed GMO feed full of pesticides and herbicides, apart from antibiotics – all the things that destroy our digestive systems! Even if the price is twice as high, per egg it doesn't really matter – or you have to eat one egg instead of two.

Avoid super pasteurized products - the normal is bad enough. If you have a chance, buy raw, organic dairy.

In the fish department, buy only wild caught fish or fish "farmed with awareness."

Seafood from Asia is always farmed and not with good feed either. They have a lot of foreign additives in them and the fish farms are very dirty and polluting.

Buy organic, grass fed beef and poultry, or at least hormone free and antibiotic free animal proteins. They are still fed with GMO corn and the pesticides that come with it.

If you make or buy bone broth, make sure it is organic or it will contain lead, together with other undesired impurities. The best is to make your own, either from grass fed beef or organic chicken.

For vegetables – always try to buy organic.

Don't buy fruit juices! They have added sugars, sometimes color and preservatives! Make your own vegetable juice! You can add an apple or a couple of carrots to sweeten it up and maybe a couple of drops of stevia.

Start to become conscious and aware about what your autistic child eats that leads to behaviors like temper tantrums.

I didn't say it was easy. Especially if you have been on the SAD diet (Standard American Diet), but then, on the other hand, you will see faster results.

Avoid the center aisles, where you find all the processed foods and desserts, cookies, sweets, and all the things you will have to stop eating.

Avoid store-bought salad dressing, ketchup, and mustard. Salad dressing is the easiest thing to make, just mix lemon and olive oil, some salt and maybe organic mustard. You can make a larger batch and have it for the whole week or more.

Ketchup has HFCS, corn syrup, and sugar as ingredients number one, two and three. Maybe water is number one, but you get it.

This goes for everything sauce-like, if not organic. You really have to read labels.

Stay away from Nutella, jellies, jams, preserves and fruit spreads. They are full of corn syrup, HFCS, and sugar, all together. Strawberry jam, for example, has strawberries, which are among the most toxic and sprayed berries on the planet. Then add all the sugar – 12 grams of sugar per tablespoon of jam - what do you think of that? HFCS and corn syrup of course are GMO foods and so is beet sugar.

Stay away from wheat. If gluten intolerant, you have to stay away from most grains, but most are sensitive to the wheat and the toxins in wheat.

If you buy bread, get organic bread, made from something not wheat and read the label so wheat is not mixed in there.

I know, there is a lot to learn, but write a food diary for your autistic child to see reactions, when and how long after eating for starters.

Don't stress yourself out in the beginning. Do one thing at a time and see how it goes.

To help lessen your child's behavior problems and other life challenges, I talked about the importance of The Allergy Kit. With The Allergy Kit, coupled with diet and nutrition, you can really see your child begin to thrive again. In the next chapter, I'm going to walk you through the different types of diets that, when combined with the kit, can help your child.

Diet and Nutrition

Nutrition is key in your child's ability to thrive on all levels – growing, physically and mentally. Having a lot of symptoms and reactions from foods that often are so unthinkably related to food, that when you start a food diary, writing down how they feel on waking up, after food, how they behave during the day and anything different – even for the better – will give you a lot to think about!

I am sure you will have big AHA's, connecting foods and reactions!

Gluten-Free Casein-Free Diet (GFCF)

Regardless of allergy test results, this is a great place to start. Almost everyone who gets on this diet has results, some great and others just a little, but so many kids show improvement, so it is worth a try.

Wheat, rye, barley, oats have the gluten protein and so does millet, even though the latter seems to be less harmful.

Quinoa is a seed so by definition, gluten-free, but they may be cross-pollinated and maybe have some gluten. It should be cooked in a pressure cooker to be absorbed better when eaten.

Unfortunately, wheat is hidden in so many products, so it is important to read labels. If you don't have your child stay away from wheat 100 percent, you will not get the result you're looking for! Some children start talking after avoiding all foods with wheat.

Symptoms of gluten intolerance can be diarrhea or constipation, while the casein allergy seems to cause more constipation. Vomiting clear mucus is a common sign of casein intolerance, and growing pains in the legs can also be due to casein allergy. Casein is the protein found in dairy.

Other symptoms of gluten/casein allergy can be high pain tolerance and self-injury.

GFCF diet is a great starting point and foundation for most diets. It is great to do while you're treating your child with The Allergy Kit. Doing both to start with may improve your child's symptoms of diarrhea and constipation and may also reduce many cognitive and behavioral habits!

There are many hidden sources of gluten and casein in all kinds of products, so it can be very difficult to eliminate it totally from the diet, and it is important to make the diet as effective as possible. Eliminating the allergies will be very helpful, since the reactions will be much less or none at all. But it is still important to stay away from these products, since the most important thing is to heal the gut from these inflammatory foods.

GFCF, Gluten-Free/Casein-Free diet is not necessarily healthy. Lots of baked goods made with other kinds of flour, are not only more processed than the original, they are also loaded with sugars and artificial sweeteners and they are very addicting. But try to put these kids on a low sugar diet.

Unfortunately, when dairy and wheat are eliminated from the diet, you also lose some nutrients. I recommend my patients start taking JuicePlus+, which is made from raw, fresh fruits and vegetables. The calcium from dark green veggies are better absorbed than calcium from milk, and often, since the body craves what we eat, they start to want to eat vegetables!

Whey has lactoferrin, a precursor to glutathione, which always is lacking in ASD kids. It's been known ASD kids can't transform lactoferrin into glutathione. That could be why they are so low in glutathione, and why they often crave milk!

Glutathione is very important for antioxidant production and specifically for a healthy brain. It is also important for detoxification, which is so difficult for children with ASD, so they may need to take it as a supplement.

It can often be very difficult to put an ASD child on the GFCF diet because that's all they want to eat! It can be the cause to a lot of fights over food cravings for pizza, bread, and milk– the foods that are harmful to them. As a parent, however, you have to stand your ground! You're the boss, not the child, and, after all, you are doing this for their health and well-being!

I know parents who say it is too expensive and that it is too hard. "I will never be able to get my child off of wheat and processed foods, since that is all they want." You have to insist and keep doing it. If they don't want to eat anything else, then they can't eat anything. They will not starve to death, believe me.

You also have to stay away from soy and MSG. Some parents think they can give them soymilk, but no, they can't have that either! It is a GMO food, an endocrine disruptor, and a highly reactive product!

MSG totally plays with the neurons in the brain and not in a good way!

There are so many testimonials from parents who have put their kids on the GFCF diet and have miraculous results in a very short time! They start to have direct eye contact with their parents and even with strangers, and they start talking and playing. They get potty-trained.

According to an Autism Research Institute survey, a gluten and casein-free diet is helpful for about 65 percent of children with ASD, and sometimes it helps for a short time and then it stops. It is probably best to eliminate first one, say wheat and gluten, and then casein to see what happens. If you keep them on milk, make sure it is raw milk.

A food diary is very helpful. It is difficult to remember what kind of food they ate in hindsight, and how they felt overall; so writing it down helps a lot.

Everything never works for everybody. Try it out as best as you can and check for reactions, setbacks, or regressions and go from there.

GFCF diet can be very effective if followed with awareness. It may be difficult in the beginning, but when you see the results you will be very pleased.

Before you remove anything and get yourself and your family upset, introduce GFCF alternatives. If they're used to eating pancakes and waffles, try GF waffles and rice pasta.

Eliminate milk and milk products for a couple of weeks, and then start them on raw, unpasteurized milk and yogurt.

Eliminate wheat for up to six months, so the gut can heal – wheat is a very inflammatory food and not good if they have gut problems.

Avoid sugars and sweeteners like the plague. That can be very difficult but try some fruit instead but not too much – they have sugar too!

The GFCF diet is the beginning. Sometimes it is the only diet the child needs, and other times you have to try some of the other diets, depending on the candida, other allergies, etc., but everything starts in the gut. Take a deep breath and go ahead. It could be the beginning of a new life.

Specific Carbohydrate Diet (SCD)

The SCD diet was introduced by Dr. Merrill Patterson Haas and Dr. Sidney Valentine Haas in the early 1950s, when they published a book titled *Management of Celiac Disease*.

The book was directed to the medical community, documenting hundreds of cases of celiac disease as well as cases of cystic fibrosis of the pancreas, but it was not taken up by other doctors.

Their approach was dietary, using a well-balanced, so-called "normal" diet, Remember, this was in the 1950s, before fast food entered the picture. This diet was specific as to the types of sugars and starches allowed.

Elaine Gotchall took her very sick daughter to Dr. Merrill Haas in 1958, after having been diagnosed as having an incurable ulcerative colitis, and surgery was inevitable according to her doctor. The girl was 8 years old.

Dr. Haas saved her life without surgery, only using his Specific Carbohydrate Diet, and Elaine Gotchall started to study with him until his death at 93 years old. She then, at the age of 47, went to study at the university, and received her bachelor's degree from the Department of Biology at Montclair State College in 1973 in biology, nutritional biochemistry, and cellular biology.

From then, until her death, she worked and helped tens of thousands of people with digestive problems and children with ASD.

The SCD diet is very effective for ASD children and is recognized from Defeat Autism Now! (DAN!) doctors, who claim that the SCD diet is the best treatment they have found for many children with ASD.

The principle is that some individuals can't digest carbohydrates, maybe due to inflammation in the intestines and to food allergies. This leads to destruction of good bacteria and enzymes, preventing absorption of carbohydrates, creating fermentation in the GI tract, with further chemical injuries from microbial toxins, acids, and the presence of undigested food in the stool.

How Does It Work?

Research indicates that starches and certain sugars feed microbes, such as bacteria, yeast, and fungi. These harmful microbes in the intestinal tract cause GI problems, autism, Alzheimer's, depression, ADHD, ADD, and other illnesses.

SCD diet eliminates these microbes by starving them, while nourishing the body. As the body heals the gut/brain connection is repaired.

How Is It Different from Gluten-Free Casein-Free (GFCF)?

You can remain GFCF on SCD. SCD is gluten-free, but does not allow starch and sugar. SCD includes dairy that is virtually lactose free and contains denatured casein. However, dairy foods are not mandatory on SCD.

Pam Ferro, of The Gottschall Autism Center and Hopewell Clinic, says the first three months for ASD children should be dairy-free. The majority of ASD children begin SCD without dairy, and many successfully integrate dairy back into their diet after some healing occurs.

How Successful Is Specific Carbohydrate Diet (SDC)?

Anecdotal reports indicate a success rate of 80-85 percent. With guidance, this rate increases.

Pam Ferro, R.N. of The Gottschall Center, reports an amazing success rate with the children she has been treating. Parents and teachers of autistic children on SCD report a change in their attitude, increase in skills and responsiveness. In some of these cases, it occurs only a few weeks after beginning the diet. Many children recover with SCD. As one mother has said, "When you see them emerge, the true child, with a loving personality, like an iridescent butterfly breaking out of its cocoon, well, that's why we all persevere."

What Kind of Food Is Required?

SCD uses healthy nutritious meat, fish, poultry, fruits, vegetables, cheeses, honey, nuts, and milk that are incubated into yogurt to remove the lactose and denature the casein. These natural foods are used to create kid-friendly recipes such as ketchup, crackers, cookies etc.

Support

To receive help with SCD, you can join the SCD children's list, *Pecanbread*. The Pecan Bread Yahoo group provides help, encouragement, and motivation from Veterans of SCD and from other families doing the SCD. Help is available from SCD individual counselors.

Common Questions from Parents about SCD

Q: My child is a picky eater. Can they still do SCD?

A: Picky eating may be a sign of starch addiction which many children lose after they do SCD.

Q: My child is allergic to nuts, eggs, and dairy.

A: SCD can be implemented despite these restrictions. As the SCD heals the gut, many allergies and sensitivities go away.

Q: My child does not have any GI symptoms. Can they still benefit from SCD?

A: SCD is a balanced, healthy, nutritional diet and generally beneficial to overall health. Many parents of ASD children find that despite having no obvious GI symptoms, SCD helps their children behaviorally. Many symptoms seem natural and parents don't think of them as obvious GI problems, but bloating and gas are symptoms, too.

Treating with The Allergy Kit greatly helps the outcome using this diet!

What's for Dinner (And Breakfast, Lunch and Snacks)?

There are hundreds of free recipes on the Internet and a number of terrific SCD Cookbooks. See **Further Reading** for references to recipes and other websites with helpful information.

SCD is the second most common ASD diet. It seems to be very helpful when the child has chronic diarrhea or inflamed gut.

What if the GFCF Diet doesn't work?

Does other food bother them, like grains or meat?

What about nuts?

The GFCF is very useful in reducing inflammation caused by food allergies in ASD kids, including reducing chronic diarrhea when the bowels are very inflamed. However, ASD kids are often allergic to even some of the foods in the GFCF diet. Therefore, this diet works very well together with The Allergy Kit, which can help eliminate those food allergies.

Some children respond very well to this kind of diet, but it is difficult to follow, especially in the beginning, until you learn what foods are allowed (legal) and which are not (illegal).

I recommend the book *Breaking the Vicious Cycle: Intestinal Health Through Diet* .There is a lot of information that explains about which foods are "legal and illegal."

This diet also allows raw dairy. I would suggest you wait before you use dairy, and I also insist that you eliminate allergies first with The Allergy Kit.

Raw dairy can be very nutritious if they can tolerate it. The pasteurization of milk makes it chemically totally different from raw milk and doesn't have the benefits at all. Nowadays there is high pasteurization of milk, so it can last for months! Don't go for it – it is not milk anymore.

Raw milk can help asthma. Yogurt has many beneficial ingredients that are good for the digestion but be careful in the beginning. Don't start adding even raw milk in the beginning of the SCD diet.

Whey is helpful for the glutathione production that is so important in detoxification; thus raw milk is important.

If there are no sensitivities, these are **some of the allowed SCD foods** according to Julie Matthews book, *Nourishing Hope for Autism*:

- Meat
- Eggs
- Natural cheeses
- Homemade yogurt
- Non-starchy veggies
- Some beans: dried white (navy) beans, lentils, split peas, lima beans

- Fruit and 100% fruit juice not from concentrate
- Nuts
- Honey
- Nut milk
- Olive oil
- Coconut oil
- Organic corn oil
- Spices, except curry and mixtures like apple pie spice
- Ghee

Foods to avoid

- Corn
- Potatoes
- Grains
- Products made from grains or starches
- Beans
- Soy
- Molasses
- Corn syrup artificial sweeteners including Splenda
- Garlic or onion powder
- Cornstarch, arrowroot powder, tapioca, agar-agar
- Pectin
- Jellies and jams

- Chocolate or carob
- Ketchup
- Baking powder (baking soda is fine)

The SCD diet uses the principle that some individuals cannot digest carbohydrates, probably due to damage to the mucosa of the small intestine and inflammation of the gut. This produces yeast overgrowth, as they feed on unabsorbed complex sugars creating a "vicious cycle."

The Body Ecology Diet

The Body Ecology Diet was developed by Donna Gates. This is probably the best diet if your child has candida, which seems to be the case in 100 percent of the ASD kids. Almost everybody today has been treated for some type of infection, whether for an ear infection or strep throat (often stemming from an allergy to milk) and has been given one or more courses of antibiotics. So therefore, candida overgrowth is very common in the American population and all over the world where antibiotics are used.

Antibiotics are the real culprits when it comes to candida, since the antibiotics kill everything – both good and bad bacteria, so the bad bacteria get the upper hand. Since the bad bacteria need sugar, starches, and sugary foods to survive and proliferate, they will call for this in the form of cravings. And this is what we see in these kids and grownups, too for that matter – sugar cravings – big time!

To handle this, the "bad" bacteria have to be starved, so there can be a balance between the good and the bad for healing to take place.

This is a so-called food combination diet, which means that you eat meat with non-starchy veggies and salads, and starches with veggies and salads, but you can't eat meat and starches, like potatoes or rice, together.

The same goes for fruits. You cannot eat acid fruits together with sweet fruits, for example, strawberries with bananas or blueberries!

The reason for this is that these combinations ferment in the digestive tract and instead of the nutrients being absorbed, they rot in the intestines and cause bloating, pain, foul smelling gas, and diarrhea or constipation, just to mention a few of the inconveniences.

Eating fruits after a meal consisting of animal protein is also a no-no, since the fruits only need about 15 minutes to pass through the digestive system while the protein needs hours. So, the fruit will sit on top of the longer-to-digest foods, trying to pass through, causing gas and discomfort.

You can't have sugars either! This is probably the hardest part for the ASD kids and adults with candida, but the idea is to starve the candida bacteria.

Allowable fruit consumption is also low, since many of them are very sugary.

How do you know if your child has candida? You can look at their tongue and if there is a white, often thick coating, this is a sign of candida.

You can also do the so-called spit test. You ask the child to spit in a glass of water and see what happens to the saliva. If it "grows" long strings toward the bottom of the glass, they have candida.

Candida per se has a long array of symptoms, both neurological, emotional, and physical. Candida is very common in ASD, mostly due to antibiotics.

Since candida thrives on certain bacteria and needs sugars and sugary food to reproduce, it will always crave these foods. It is like an addiction and the diet can often be difficult to handle, especially in the beginning. The child will not be happy when you change their diet and the hardest thing is to be strong and show who the boss is! When the candida bacteria start to get starved, they will scream for sugar, because they are dying! They, like everything else, want to live.

Sometimes there are so called die-off reactions. They may get headaches, feel nauseous, have foul smelling gas and stools, and feel bad in general, but it will be worth the effort, even with the bad experiences.

The results will amaze you, even though it may be ugly for a few days. Just hang in there and remember there is light at the end of the tunnel.

The gut/brain barrier is well known by now. As we've already learned, the gut is called the second brain! Whatever goes on in the gut affects the brain. If there is candida, the affected person may feel spacey, may have difficulty focusing or thinking straight, have weird behavior, and a lot of gastric and digestive problems.

For best results, they may have to be on a sugar-free, antibiotic/steroids-free and immune suppressing drug-free consumption for up to six months! They have to eliminate all refined and simple sugars, malts, HFCS, corn syrup, maple syrup, chocolate, and artificial sweeteners.

Eliminate

- Eliminate foods rich in yeast and molds, like cheeses, dried foods, melons (all melons) and peanuts.
- Eliminate all kinds of fermented sauces coming in bottles: soy sauce, Worcester sauce, and anything with vinegar, like pickles.
- Try to eliminate fruits, at least in the beginning and then you can add one or two fruits a day.
- All kind of so called cold cuts, hot dogs, and processed meats.
- Eliminate everything with artificial flavor, colors, and preservatives.
- No milk or dairy.
- Can use Stevia
- They can eat organic chicken, turkey, beef and fish.
- Vegetables
- Quinoa (has to be cooked in pressure cooker)
- Some beans; black-eyed peas, garbanzo beans, lima beans, mung beans, red lentils
- White rice (easier to digest)
- No milk or dairy. Use ghee instead of butter
- Coconut oil for cooking
- Olive oil for everything else
- Some blueberries

You can add some bacteria suppressing herbs or essential oils, but consult with a practitioner or herb specialist, because you don't want to go too fast and have a die-off reaction.

You may want to add some probiotics, but same thing, go slow. Best thing is to muscle test, to make sure they can handle them. Some people are sensitive to probiotics and fermented foods, even though they desperately need them! Sometimes, giving them a very small amount at a time can help build up the good bacteria and enzymes very slowly, which can be a great help.

I suggest you read Donna Gates' book *The Body Ecology Diet*.

Nourishing Traditions/Weston Price Diet

Weston Price, a dentist, travelled around the world in the 1930s and 1940s, to find out if there was any connection between health and nutrition. He visited indigenous cultures and found different diets depending on their environment.

Some were plant-based and others animal-based, but since this was long before McDonalds and Burger King, no processed food whatsoever was consumed.

He found these people to be perfectly healthy, with perfect, straight teeth, perfect bones, no heart attacks or cancer, and great skin, to mention just a few indications of great health.

Now if we go back to these same places, we find that all this great health is gone. People have very bad teeth, if any; when a little older, their face bones have changed, and the teeth are no longer straight. They have heart attacks, diabetes, and everything else we have in the West, since they now are consuming sodas, canned food, and white bread – all the "good" civilized habits were introduced.

The following is an overview of what the Price diet focuses on, but remember - it has to be organic! This diet works very well if allergies are eliminated first, since this diet consists of allergen foods.

- Animal foods and fats
- Dairy and butter - raw and unprocessed
- Sprouted grains and beans
- Stocks and broths
- Coconuts and coconut oil
- Salads and veggies
- Nothing processed - that didn't exist in Dr. Price's time!

The main focus in this diet is natural, organic, clean foods. It works very well when eliminating allergies first. It is very simple, really. The main thing is that the food is organic; the dairy has to be raw. It seems most people with milk allergies are fine with raw milk and only react to the pasteurized milk, which is now ultra-pasteurized.

The pasteurization process totally changes the chemical properties in milk - even though it looks like milk, smells like milk, and tastes like milk – it is not milk anymore!

You can learn more by reading the book *Nourishing Traditions* by Sally Fallon.

So, Now What Do We Eat?

Yes, I know. It looks difficult – you think there is nothing left to eat! But stay calm because there are still many food choices.

You will have to start cooking, though, if you didn't before, because what you have to stay away from is processed, store-bought food or food from some fast food restaurant.

And yes, I know it is more expensive to buy organic food, and it does take more time to go to stores that sell organic foods, and it also takes more time to go to the market, where you can find both organic and local produce, but it will be worth it.

Maybe you can make it fun by going with the whole family! Sometimes being or doing something together can satisfy the kids' wishes.

Not every diet fits everybody. There are more diets available than I have included in this book, but these suggestions are good to start with.

If your child has some specific reactions to some other foods, they may be sensitive to foods high in oxalates or phenols, for example.

Some common foods high in oxalate are:

- Greens: spinach, Swiss chard, beet greens, parsley
- Nuts and seeds, almonds, cashews, peanuts
- Legumes: soybean and most beans

- Grains: wheat, spelt, kamut, Buckwheat, amaranth
- Fruits: blackberries, raspberries, gooseberries, currants, kiwifruit, figs, star fruit.
- Vegetables: celery, beets, okra, sweet potato, rhubarb
- Other: cocoa, chocolate, black tea.

Reactions and symptoms from eating high oxalate foods are often: pain, stomach pain, headache, low energy, urinary tract infections, poor motor skills, and more.

If they are allergic to phenols, common in artificial colors and additives, and in some fruits and smells, the reaction is often immediate or within 20 minutes, and can show up as hyperactivity, red cheeks and ears, and many more. I think problems with touch and noise can come from this kind of sensitivity, too.

Candida is often present, and they often crave the high oxalate foods.

After treating with The Allergy Kit, they can have eggs, which makes breakfasts so much easier.

Growing your own veggies is a great way to encourage your kids like to eat them! An easy way to do that is with the Tower Garden from JuicePlus+! Check it out – it is easy, doesn't need any dirt or a big place!

Other Diets

Many children are allergic or sensitive to salicylates - the substance in Aspirin, found in the willow tree. It occurs in many plants and fruits, veggies, and herbs. They are also created synthetically, like in Bayer's aspirin pills and found in many other medicines, perfumes, and preservatives.

They act as a natural immune hormone and preservatives to protect the plants from diseases, insects, harmful bacteria, and fungi.

Symptoms are many and some of the physical symptoms are:

- Itchy skin, hives or rashes
- Stomach pain/upset stomach
- Asthma
- Headaches
- Swelling of hands and feet
- Breathing difficulties
- Bed wetting
- Mouth ulcers or raw hot red rash around mouth
- Persistent cough
- Frequent need to urinate/urgency to pass water
- Wheezing
- Changes in skin color/skin discoloration
- Swelling of eyelids, face and lips
- Fatigue
- Sore, itchy, puffy, or burning eyes
- Watering eyes
- Anaphylaxis (this is very rare, but deadly)
- Sinusitis

Mental and Behavioral Symptoms:

- Hyperactivity
- Poor concentration
- Cognitive and perceptual disorders
- Depression
- ADD and ADHD
- Irritability
- Central nervous system depression
- Accident prone
- Anxiety
- Anger for no apparent reason
- Behavioral problems
- Blankness
- Brain fogging
- Changes in handwriting
- Clumsiness
- Confusion

As you can see, there are a lot of reactions and the above mentioned are just a few, but they may explain why your child behaves in a certain way at certain times. The reactions can also be delayed, which makes it even more difficult to understand what's happening.

Histamine and Amine Intolerance

People who are salicylate intolerant can also develop an amine sensitivity or histamine intolerance. You can find histamine and the similar amine substances, occurring naturally in a variety of foods, like aged cheese, processed and aged meats, citrus fruits, soy sauce, and sauerkraut, to mention a few.

They especially develop from the breakdown of protein and fermentation that occurs during food processing and that's why some people, when eating the healthy, fermented foods, often recommended, can't tolerate the sauerkraut or kefir!

It has to do with the sulfation, that doesn't process normally in ASD kids and people. Sulfation is the ability to utilize sulfate in a wide variety of biochemical processes, and also the name of phase two detoxification pathway in the liver. It is involved in enzyme, protein, and tissue synthesis, as well as in production of bile acids, digestion, detoxifications, and cellular respiration. It is also one of the most abundant minerals in the body. Kind of important, don't you think?

Fermented foods include cheeses, especially aged and meats that are too old (leftovers and cooked too long), pickles, and yogurt, to mention a few.

Possible symptoms include: flushing, sweating, heart palpitation, headaches, itching, rashes, diarrhea or constipation, abdominal cramps, asthma, and more.

Phenol is another organic chemical compound, like salicylates, present in many foods, food dyes, and additives.

Almost all foods have phenols in different amounts and seem to affect children on the ASD; it has to do with the faulty sulfation so many suffer from. Treating with The Allergy Kit is very important to help with the sensitivity to these organic compounds that have so many negative reactions.

Phenols, salicylates, food dyes, and additives are problems that can be addressed after the gluten-free/casein-free (GFCF) diet has been started. Generally, it is recommended for parents to address foods high in phenols, salicylates, and additives about two to six months after starting the GFCF or other similar diet. Observing the child and writing a diary can be very helpful, and in the case of seeing some definite reactions after consuming specific foods, eliminate that food.

Almost all foods have phenols, but in different amounts. A child with low PST (phenol sulfur transferase) will have trouble processing foods high in phenols, so reduce or avoid eating foods high in phenols so their body does not overload when trying to process the phenols it will ingest anyway.

Eating foods high in phenol or foods containing salicylates and/or additives may experience some of these negative side effects:

- laughing at inappropriate times (at night or when something is not funny)
- strange rashes that appear on the body
- erratic behaviors and moods
- self-stimulatory behaviors
- waking up in the middle of the night
- having a difficult time with their stools (constipation, diarrhea, and/or undigested foods in the stool)
- headaches

These symptoms could also be due to autism or other medical issues. Some experience some of the issues above and others not.

Many families with children on the ASD found that by eliminating or greatly reducing the ingestion of phenols, symptoms went away, only to return when there was a forbidden food infraction.

There are hundreds of products that contain high levels of phenols and salicylates, and countless food sources with dyes and additives. Interestingly, food dyes, tomatoes, apples, peanuts, bananas, oranges, cocoa, red grapes, vanilla extract, all kinds of natural and artificial flavors, and colorings all contain levels of phenols and salicylates.

Supplements

ASD children have vitamin and mineral deficiencies due to their damaged gut, so they cannot absorb the nutrients from foods.

Being picky eaters doesn't help and this is where lifestyle changes are so important!

By eliminating allergies with the kit is a big help since it helps both with sugar and food cravings, which in turn will help to heal the gut and nutrient absorption.

I don't recommend many supplements for them, first because their bodies don't absorb them and that can make them feel sick. Second, there is a lot of work to do just to feed them without making them take a lot of supplements, and third, it makes them even more toxic!

I recommend JuicePlus+, because it is normally very well absorbed and digested, and it is whole food in capsules that also can be opened and put into a drink or spread over the food.

For younger children or for the ones that won't take the capsules or the powder, there are chewables. They have very little sugar in fruit juice form and can be given as a little snack for the sweet tooth, without jeopardizing when candida is present, which is most cases.

ASD children also often have an imbalance between copper and zinc. The best thing is to have them tested by a functional practitioner or doctor.

Pumpkin seeds, for example, are rich in zinc, and when roasted are a great snack!

Fermented food is very good because of its great content of enzymes. Half a cup of raw sauerkraut, eaten cold not to destroy them, has more enzymes than a whole bottle of probiotics.

Some people can't handle enzymes due to an allergy to them, but that can be remedied with, you guessed it: The Allergy Kit!

Then, after having gone through the basic treatments with the kit, you start by giving them a very small amount of, for example, sauerkraut.

It is very easy to prepare fermented foods and Donna Gates has several how to videos on YouTube, or you can get her book, *The Body Ecology Diet*, which is all about her diet The Body Ecology Diet, or BED.

She has many suggestions about different fermented foods, both vegetable, dairy, and coconut kefir and much more!

Vitamin C is a vitamin that is essential for the body and ASD kids are often low in this. It is not supplemented with orange juice. Some believe that is the best way, but it is not.

Drinking the juice, pressed days or weeks before buying it, with sugars and preservatives, maybe color added, makes the sugar go directly into the blood, creating a sugar spike and giving the pancreas a hard time to try to regulate the insulin and blood sugar.

When you eat a fruit, there is a delayed sugar reaction which is much healthier, but not enough to supplement the vitamin C.

You can buy vitamin C in powder form and mix it in a drink, maybe with some vegetable juice, or you can go to Designs for Health to get some of the most commonly needed supplements.

Just remember to go slowly in the beginning.

Again, keep a diary – every day – to be able to see what reactions they have to what, how they recuperate, how their appetite and cravings change, how their sleep is, and everything else.

Mineral Deficiencies

The Importance of Magnesium

Magnesium also plays an important role in ensuring the proper function of calcium. Many people suffer from a magnesium deficiency. Magnesium and vitamin K have a symbiotic relationship, each improving the other's ability to improve health. You can choose to use magnesium citrate or magnesium threonate supplements. In addition to oral supplements, you can improve your child's magnesium intake transdermal through oils which can be applied to the skin and/or poured into bath water.

You can easily add more magnesium to your family's daily diet. Foods high in magnesium include bananas; figs; dark, leafy greens; oatmeal; quinoa; brown rice; lentils and beans. Sea vegetables, such as kelp, dulse, and nori, although less popular in the U.S. than in many Asian cultures, also provide an excellent source of magnesium.

There is a particularly strong connection between magnesium deficiency and the brain. As Dr. Carolyn Dean writes in *The Magnesium Miracle*, "Magnesium permits calcium to enter a nerve cell to allow electrical transmission along the nerves to and from the brain. Even our thoughts, via brain neurons, are dependent on magnesium."

Signs of magnesium deficiency include:

- Restlessness, can't keep still, body rocking
- Grinding teeth
- Hiccups
- Noise sensitivity
- Poor attention span and concentration
- Irritable
- Aggressive and ready to explode and
- Easily stressed

Parents of children with ASD will readily recognize these symptoms.

Magnesium Absorption

Children with autism tend to have difficulty absorbing nutrients. Magnesium absorption in particular can be difficult because magnesium from food sources and/or orally administered supplements depends on intestinal health for successful absorption. Leaky gut syndrome and other intestinal problems so common in autism and similar syndromes interfere with the ability of children with ASD to absorb the magnesium, which can help them.

Magnesium's role in helping the body eliminate toxins

Magnesium is very important for phase one detoxification because it, along with other minerals like zinc, displaces toxic heavy metals from the body. Magnesium is a crucial factor in the natural self-cleansing and detoxification responses of the body.

Zinc and Copper

Children with ASD often exhibit an imbalance in zinc and copper levels. What is important here is the ratio between the two. Most children on the ASD are zinc deficient but have excessively high levels of copper, which is very important to find out and rectify.

Balancing Zinc and Copper Levels

Health experts estimate that at least one in ten Americans fail to consume enough zinc in their diets. Zinc is actually present in a wide variety of protein containing foods. Animal products such as red meat, egg yolk, organ meats, and seafood, as well as certain nuts, seeds, beans, and cereal grains contain zinc. The recommended daily allowance for zinc is currently set at 8-11 mg, which is certainly achievable from food sources. Yet, the issue lies not simply with crude zinc intake, but also in how accessible the sources are by the body. Plant sources of zinc are bound by anti-nutrients like phytic acid. These interfere with zinc absorption.

One reason for zinc deficiency could be from the nutrients in foods that one is allergic to and the body can't absorb. This could be eliminated by clearing the allergies with the The Allergy Kit.

Beef or lamb, liver, and oysters are by far the best sources of this powerful mineral, with four times the absorption rate of their plant counterparts, and a balanced ratio of other trace minerals. However, in our fat-phobic, grain-chomping society, people tend to avoid these zinc-rich foods. During the Paleolithic era, humans may have consumed an average of 50 mg of zinc per day from whole food sources. Unfortunately, excess sugar intake, alcohol, stress, heart disease, and infection further suppress levels of this critical nutrient. This is yet another reason to avoid processed foods!

To be able to absorb zinc, it may be a good idea to clear any allergy/sensitivity to zinc. By absorbing more zinc, the ratio zinc/copper will rectify itself.

I presented different diets, because each one addresses different symptoms that your child may exhibit. Just remember, it is important to use The Allergy Kit along with the diet, whichever you choose according to their symptoms.

Lifestyle

I t may be difficult but very worthwhile. You and your family may be resistant to change in food choices and to really change lifestyle and learn, not only about food and nutrition, but also about things that can be very abrasive to your child, like perfumes, air fresheners, detergents and house cleaners, to mention a few.

My hope and expectation are that once you get a handle on it, you and everybody in your family, including your autistic child will feel so good, that you embrace the new knowledge.

Cleaning up the House

The next thing to do is to go through all the cleaning supplies, detergents, clothes softener, window cleaners, and air fresheners – everything you use that has a smell/scent!

Haven't you found sometimes you pass a person and the smell from the detergent in their clothes is so strong that you start to sneeze?

So many people react to different smells and start sneezing and getting a stuffy nose. For ASD kids, it is much more serious. They can have all kinds of reactions from asthma attacks to total meltdowns, seizures, stop talking, and many more.

At times, you don't think about what it is that is changing your child, especially not in the beginning of changing foods and lifestyle. When they often have reactions and/or have them all the time and you don't know why, smells can be a big culprit!

House cleaning is as important as the lifestyle change and cleaning up the diet!

After WWII, there was a surge in the chemical industry, and the environment has since been flooded with new chemicals. Over 80,000 chemicals are used in everyday products! They are everywhere! In the plastic we handle, in our water and food, and in the air. Chemicals are impossible to avoid. There are no regulations or safety rules to find out if these chemicals are safe to use. Chemicals are considered safe until proven otherwise.

Researchers are now suspecting the use of industrial chemicals gives rise to lower IQs, cancer, and reproductive problems, as some of the many disorders and problems we have today and are seeing more and more every day.

Without adequate testing – are we the guinea pigs in a huge experiment?

Chemical pollution starts in the womb. Mothers are exposed to these toxins and inadvertently pass them through to their unborn baby. There is no way around it.

The dangers of mercury and lead have been known for decades, but there are many other chemicals around now whose side effects are not known.

There are toxins in cans, bisphenol A (BPA), and even if the companies say there is none, that it has been taken out, there are other phenols in there that they don't mention, and there is no research on what these do.

There are toxins in all kind of cosmetics, hair sprays, perfumes, lipsticks, and the list goes on.

Lots of the chemicals are endocrine disruptors, and they come in many forms and things.

Furniture and mattresses are treated with a flame-retardant chemical by law. Other endocrine disruptors are plastics of all kinds.

Plastics are not safe! Babies chew on their plastic toys, many mothers heat food and even baby food and formula in plastic in the microwave – a big no-no! This makes these "fake" hormones leak out into the food causing a lot of problems.

Girls are going into puberty from 8 years of age or younger. Boys may have undescended testicles or digenesis (the urethra doesn't exit at the tip of the penis).

Low sperm count is now common, and testicular cancer has gone up 50 percent, starting in much younger men already in their 30s.

IQ in children has gone down, and there are less *gifted* children than before.

Some chemicals store in the body for decades, others have a short-lived effect, but we may be exposed all the time.

Water bottles leak out these estrogen-like hormones and it affects all of us - not only humans, but animals too.

Did you think about air fresheners? Totally toxic!

Alligators in Florida have messed up sex organs – are they females or males? The same with fish in areas where there are a lot of chemicals being disposed into the water from factories.

Cookware

Teflon and other non-stick cookware expel a poisonous gas when heated, especially on high heat, so when frying food this is very dangerous and many people, not only ASD kids, are very sensitive to this! The best is ceramic coated cookware, of course, more expensive, but totally worth it!

Dr. Mercola, who has the world's biggest health newsletter, couldn't understand why he felt bad when he ate at home, until he realized that it was the nonstick cookware that made him sick. When he got rid of it, he immediately felt better!

Quick Cures for Stress

There are several quick exercises you can do for yourself or for your child that will help calm down, reduce stress, and ground the person.

Body Talk Tapping for Mom

This exercise takes a bit more time, so it may not be best for an "in the moment" need. However, when you have a free moment, you might want to gift yourself with the benefits of using this technique just for yourself so you feel better.

In this exercise, we will be tapping on all parts of the brain and the heart complex.

1. Start by putting your hand over the lower back of the head. While holding this part with one hand, use the other hand to tap in a circular motion around the tip-top of the head.

   Inhale as you tap on the top, then exhale as you tap on your heart area.

   Repeat this step two times.

2. Move hand up to the next area. We want to eventually cover all parts of the brain. And tap again in a circular motion. Inhale as you tap on the top, then exhale as you tap on your heart area.

   Repeat this step two times.

3. Move hand forward again. While holding this part with one hand, use the other hand to tap in a circular motion around the tip-top of the head.

   Inhale as you tap on the top, then exhale as you tap on your heart area.

   Repeat this step two times.

4. Move forward to top of the head. And tap again in a circular motion. Inhale as you tap on the top, then exhale as you tap on your heart area.

   Repeat this step two times.

5. Move hand to the forehead. While holding this part with one hand, use the other hand to tap in a circular motion around the tip top of the head.

   Inhale as you tap on the top, then exhale as you tap on your heart area.

   Repeat this step two times.

6. Move hand to the left side of the head. While holding this part with one hand, use the other hand to tap in a circular motion around the tip top of the head.

   Inhale as you tap on the top, then exhale as you tap on your heart area.

   Repeat this step two times.

7. 7. Move hand to right side of head. While holding this part with one hand, use the other hand to tap in a circular motion around the tip top of the head.

   Inhale as you tap on the top, then exhale as you tap on your heart area.

   Take a deep breath!

Emotional Freedom Technique (EFT) Tapping

Start with the karate set-up.

First decide what you want to say, for example:

1. Even though I am exhausted and don't know what to do, I deeply and completely love and accept myself just the way I am.

2. Even though I am exhausted and don't know what to do, I deeply and completely love and accept myself, no matter what,

   Then, tap with the tip of the fingers on the right (or the left) hand, on the side of the left (or the right) hand, while you say the above sentences with intention and as if you mean it, for a couple of minutes.

Then tap on acupuncture points on the face and upper body:

They are presented below in the exact order in which they should be tapped.

1. Top of the Head (TH)

With fingers back-to-back down the center of the skull, while you're saying: I am totally exhausted.

2. Eyebrow (EB)

Just above and to one side of the nose, at the beginning of the eyebrow, while you're saying: I am totally exhausted.

3. Side of the Eye (SE)

On the bone bordering the outside corner of the eye, while you're saying: I am totally exhausted.

4. Under the Eye (UE)

On the bone under an eye about one inch below your pupil, while you're saying: I am totally exhausted.

5. Under the Nose (UN)

On the small area between the bottom of your nose and the top of your upper lip, while you're saying: I am totally exhausted.

6. Chin (CH)

Midway between the point of your chin and the bottom of your lower lip. Even though it is not directly on the point of the chin, we call it the chin point because it is descriptive enough for people to understand easily, while you're saying: I am totally exhausted.

7. Collar Bone (CB)

The junction where the sternum (breastbone), collar-bone, and the first rib meet. This is a very important point and in acupuncture is referred to as K (kidney) 27. To locate it, first place your forefinger on the U-shaped notch at the top of the breastbone (about where a man would knot his tie). From the bottom of the U, move your forefinger down toward the navel one inch, and then go to the left (or right) one inch. This point is referred to as Collar Bone even though it is not on the collarbone (or clavicle) per se, while you're saying: I am totally exhausted.

8. Under the Arm (UA)

On the side of the body, at a point even with the nipple (for men) or in the middle of the bra strap (for women). It is about four inches below the armpit, while you're saying: I am totally exhausted.

9. Wrists (WR)

The last point is the inside of both wrists, you can just tap the two wrists together, while you're saying: I am totally exhausted.

10. Repeat the same, but now you will say: I chose to let go of being tired, I chose to feel rested and happy.

EFT – Tapping for Mom

Emotional Freedom Technique (EFT) is technique that helps to balance the body's energy and bring calm to the tapper.

When we are in stressful situations, our energy stops flowing through the body as freely as it's meant to. The stressful feelings, reactions block the flow, like a hose with a kink in it. When the energy doesn't flow freely, we feel upset inside and "out of whack." When we're in this state, it's hard to think, to act, and especially to make decisions.

EFT tapping is a great way to get the energy flowing again. Think of a coin that gets stuck in a vending machine. What's the first thing you do? Kick the machine….and the product then easily flows out. That's the same with our energy system that gets kinked up. Tap on certain points of the body and the kinks come out and the energy flows.

If you're in a rush and need a "fix" right away, tap the karate chop point. This is the fleshy part of the outside of your hand that you would use to do a karate chop. You can tap this part of either hand with the fingertips of the opposite hand. OR you can use the fleshy part of one hand to "chop" the fleshy part of the other hand.

Dr. Mercola demonstrates how and where to tap. You can also watch him on *YouTube*.

The tapping points, and their abbreviations, are explained below, followed by a chart of the points. They are presented below in the exact order in which they should be tapped.

1. **Top of the Head (TH)** With fingers back-to-back down the center of the skull.

2. **Eyebrow (EB)** Just above and to one side of the nose, at the beginning of the eyebrow.

3. **Side of the Eye (SE)** On the bone bordering the outside corner of the eye.

4. **Under the Eye (UE)** On the bone under an eye about 1 inch below your pupil.

5. **Under the Nose (UN)** On the small area between the bottom of your nose and the top of your upper lip.

6. **Chin (Ch)** Midway between the point of your chin and the bottom of your lower lip. Even though it is not directly on the point of the chin, we call it the chin point because it is descriptive enough for people to understand easily.

7. **Collar Bone (CB)** The junction where the sternum (breastbone), collarbone and the first rib meet. This is a very important point and in acupuncture is referred to as K (kidney) 27. To locate it, first place your forefinger on the U-shaped notch at the top of the breastbone (about where a man would knot his tie). From the bottom of the U, move your forefinger down toward the navel 1 inch and then go to the left (or right) 1 inch. This point is referred to as Collar Bone even though it is not on the collarbone (or clavicle) per se.

8. **Under the Arm (UA)** On the side of the body, at a point even with the nipple (for men) or in the middle of the bra strap (for women). It is about 4 inches below the armpit.

9. **Wrists (WR)** The last point is the inside of both wrists.

The abbreviations for these points are summarized below in the same order as given above. It is, again, the order in which they should be tapped:

TH = Top of Head

EB = Eye Brow

SE = Side of the Eye

UE = Under the Eye

UN = Under the Nose

CH = Chin

CB = Collar Bone

UA = Under the Arm

WR = Wrists

Thymus Thump

It's difficult being a parent of a child on the autism spectrum. As the child has tantrums or hyperactive behavior, etc., it's difficult being in the middle of it. Having some easy tools to use on to get you "back to your own center of calm" are invaluable. Below are several to learn and then use when needed.

Whenever you get to your "wits' end" in the midst of your child's tantrums, etc. and feel "you're the one losing it," just take a deep breath and thump your thymus. Thump until you start to feel a bit of calmness. Your calmness will also calm your child a bit.

How to do it: Thump with your fist on the middle of your chest (on the middle of your chest bone and think about how Tarzan does it). Thump for about 20 seconds as you breathe in and out.

You will know when you have activated the thymus gland when you feel a little tingling or a sudden feeling of "joy" or "happiness" or tension relaxing.

How it works: The thymus gland lies just beneath the upper part of the breastbone in the middle of the chest. Its role is to keep your own life energy vibrating in high frequency. When the thymus gland is in harmony it does just this, but when there is emotional or physical disturbance, it can cause the thymus gland to shrink and cause depletion in this vital life energy. That's when we feel we're at our "wits' end." But thump and re-activate your own life energy. It's well worth it.

Spooning for Your Child

If a child, or any other family member for that matter, doesn't feel grounded, maybe walking on their toes a lot, or not focusing, this is a very easy trick to use.

Take a tablespoon and with the round side, run it over the naked foot, on the sole, a few times, first one foot, then the other.

This normally has a calming effect and works immediately!

These are a couple of simple treatments that can be done pretty quickly and easily. The result can be amazing!

Clearing the Body from Toxins

There are many negative offenders that we are exposed to everyday, and clearing your child's body of as many of these as possible is critical to improving their health.

In this chapter, we'll be reviewing these negative influences and giving you a background as to why they are so harmful, especially to your autistic child. I'll give you some suggestions of how to decrease further toxification, and also how to clear them from your child's body.

Some people are able to naturally remove these toxins from the body. However, others, especially autistic people, have a harder time eliminating offenders such as heavy metals.

Changing your child's diet and eliminating their allergies, as described in above chapters, will begin the body cleansing process and clear many of the toxins. However, more is required, which we will review in this chapter.

Make sure you don't skip Chapter 3 – *Where to Start*, because none of the protocols in this chapter will work if you don't clear the body of the allergies first.

Also, in Chapter 3 we looked at your child's diet and nutrition. In this chapter, we'll look at all the other factors that influence your child's health. Allergies are at the top of the list. With allergies present, more inflammation is created, more toxins are created, and it becomes a vicious cycle with the child feeling worse and worse! This is why it is so important to eliminate the allergies, doing the right kind of diet for them and detox!

Candida

Candida is bacteria that lives in the gut and normally is balanced by the good bacteria. But since almost every child gets antibiotics, sometimes several times during their childhood, plus the antibiotics in the foods they eat, candida overgrowth is extremely common. Some babies are born with it, inherited from their mother, called thrush.

Candida produces toxic byproducts that are absorbed in the intestines and then absorbed in the blood stream.

ASD kids crave sugars and sugary foods, which is both a symptom of candida and the cause of it! The candida bacteria thrive and reproduce with sugars and foods that turn into sugars, and if they don't get their "fix", the cravings can get very bad!

These symptoms in turn create hyperactivity, aggression, temper tantrums etc.

Candida also damages the immune system by destroying the enzymes necessary for proper digestion, and can even produce leaky gut, which in turn leads to food allergies.

Some of the symptoms are:

- Bloating and smelly gas
- Constipation/diarrhea, often alternating and foul smelling

- Cravings for sweets and sugary foods
- Ear/throat infections
- Food allergies
- Hyperactivity
- Eczema or rash
- Foggy thinking and disability to focus
- Obesity
- Sleep disturbances
- Stuffy nose
- Weird behavior, as if drunk or "high"

One study of preschool children indicated that one 12-ounce can of soda disrupted their performance and also increased inappropriate behavior when playing at recess.

This study also showed that grades went up when sugar was removed from their diet.

Candida overgrowth creates inflammation in the gut and damage to the GI tract, causing leaky gut, which in turn leads to allergies by the body making antibodies to the particles leaking out into the blood... where they don't belong.

The most damaging food allergies are casein in milk and the protein gliadin in wheat, that acts as an opiate in the body, not only affecting the gut, but also the brain, passing through the brain barrier.

Symptoms, apart from the ones mentioned above, can be high pain tolerance and head banging. They are trying to release something, to feel something, because they are numb from the opiate effect these foods have on them.

Eliminating the allergies to milk and wheat and grains is very helpful, but these kids should stay on a wheat-free, casein-free diet for at least six months and then try with a small amount (or muscle test), to see if they can handle it, and it *must* be organic wheat and organic, raw milk.

To eliminate the candida with diet is of utmost importance! The Body Ecology Diet, developed by Donna Gates, is the best for clearing yeast.

You have to start to eliminate the dairy and the wheat first, and then follow Donna's diet! You can find details on the diet in the previous chapter.

Mercury and Aluminum

Mercury's dangers are well established. The U.S. Environmental Protection Agency states on its website that "for fetuses, infants, and children, the primary health effect of methyl mercury is impaired neurological development."

Still, it is now recommended that pregnant women and babies under six months of age get the flu-shot – the vaccination with the highest content of thimerosal, a compound that contains mercury!

This makes no sense; especially since it has been shown that a pregnant woman receiving the flu-shot often loses her baby afterward.

Historically, the use of mercury was known as an occupational health hazard among people of the 1800s and early 1900s who used this substance to make hats. This fact was so well-known that it gave rise to the phrase "mad as a hatter." Some readers may recall Lewis Carroll's Mad Hatter character in Alice in Wonderland.

Yet our present-day risks from mercury exposure are all too often underestimated.

It is said that there is no sign of mercury after vaccinations in the blood of the receiver. But a researcher, who tested monkeys and didn't find any proof of mercury in their blood either, found that their brains were full of it in the autopsy.

The potential for mercury poisoning has increased significantly in recent years. Although mercury occurs naturally in the environment, human industrial activity has resulted in dangerous levels of this element and its compounds.

Scientists have identified mercury as a neurotoxin, meaning that mercury and its compounds can cause serious damage to the nervous system. Exposure to mercury can also have negative consequences on the functioning of the brain. Additionally, mercury has the potential to wreak havoc on other bodily systems and on our mental and emotional health.

How mercury affects the body and mind depends largely on the means of exposure. Most people have heard of the serious potential danger of broken thermometers. Many people, however, remain unaware of how easy it is to come into contact with mercury from other sources.

Nowadays, vaccines contain less thimerosal than before, but instead they have more aluminum, another neuron destroyer. Babies have no brain barrier until they are around two to three years of age and should not have any vaccines before that age! The combination of mercury and aluminum, either in the same vaccine or with vaccines together, like the flu shot

– which has thimerosal – together with any scheduled vaccination – that now has aluminum instead of mercury – is very dangerous, since the synergistic action together is even more damaging!

Dr. William Thompson was prevented from publishing results which showed that boys who had received thimerosal vaccines were developing tics. These results were developed already in 2001 when he was working at the Centers for Disease Control and Prevention (CDC) as their main researcher. The CDC personnel instead questioned whether he was psychologically stable.

Remember, the CDC is a for-profit company.

In summary, you can reduce further mercury poisoning in your child by:

- never allowing metal fillings by your child's dentist. Instead ask for resin fillings;
- avoiding further vaccinations;
- and by avoiding large fish consumption, such as tuna, more than once in a while.

There is a big difference between eating mercury and having it injected, but it is still better to avoid consumption since the toxicity is there already.

The best way to remove mercury and other heavy metals from your child's system is to use the AMD ionic foot bath for a major difference.

Aluminum has replaced mercury in vaccines, but is that really better? Aluminum is also a big threat to the brain, being a toxin to the neurons in the brain.

Autism is still on the rise in alarming speed. And it is well known that aluminum causes Alzheimer's, so why wouldn't it be causing autism, also a neurological disease?

Mold

Mold Is Poison in Our Homes and Schools

Mercury is far from the only poison at large in our modern industrial environment. Other toxic substances enter our air and even our homes through food made with preservatives; cleaning products; and gases released from plastics, carpets and many other sources.

These more recent types of health dangers have joined a pre-existing set of risks from molds caused by building deterioration. Health experts have recently come to recognize the indoor air pollution resulting from molds. Increased rain and flooding in many parts of the world have made water-damage to homes, schools, and other buildings more prevalent.

Canaries in the Coal Mine

Some of us are able to metabolize this wide array of environmental toxins better than others. For some, the toxic load takes its toll early. People with autism may be among the "canaries in the coal mine" of our modern industrial society.

There are strong indications that they have less ability than other people to metabolize environmental toxins. The difference between two siblings, one diagnosed with autism and the other not, may be that the ASD sibling has less natural ability to process and eliminate mold and other toxins.

The higher toxic load carried by people with ASD helps explain their extreme sensory sensitivity. People with autism often cannot tolerate the feeling of certain types of fabrics against their skin, or certain sounds, or specific food tastes, or textures.

Mold, the Gut and the Brain

Our gut or "second brain" contains around 100 million neurons – more than in the spinal cord or the peripheral nervous system together. It is here that serotonin, the body's natural mood elevating hormone, is created.

Research indicates that people with ASD disorders have abnormal gut flora, which not only causes GI disturbances, but also contributes to the behavioral symptoms associated with autism. Research also shows that autistic children with mold toxicity exhibit more neuropsychiatric abnormalities than other ASD kids. This is important, because it is treatable. The next section details the means for addressing mold toxicity.

Combating Mold

There are two steps for addressing the problem of mold. One, as explained below, is eliminating mold from your environment. The other is using The Allergy Kit to eliminate mold allergies. This is a very important step! Of course, we want to stay away from mold, but to get rid of the allergy is a great help, too! It is very difficult to get rid of mold allergy because mold is everywhere!

Stop Mold at the Source

The best way to completely eliminate mold toxins from the body is to avoid the source of the molds. This obviously can present a practical challenge. It can be difficult (not to mention costly) to entirely remove mold from an affected building. If a child with ASD continues to live or attend school in a building with mold, re-infection will occur. Once the source of the mold has been identified in a house or apartment, try to re-locate to a new home. If a school is the source, see if the child can transfer to another school.

Supplements, Sunshine, and Food

In sick buildings, calcium propionate is used to inhibit mold. Calcium is also important in human bodies fending off mold toxins. But rather than taking large doses of calcium, the key is to take supplements which encourage the proper functioning of calcium in the body. It is important to remember that vitamins and minerals work synergistically together to promote health.

Vitamin D

Vitamin D enables our bodies to absorb calcium. When selecting a vitamin D supplement, remember that not all supplements offer the same benefits. Look for a supplement that contains vitamin D3 along with vitamin K1 and K2. These vitamins work together as a team to ensure that your child not only gets enough calcium, but also prevents calcium build-ups in the wrong places, such as arteries and soft tissues.

Vitamin D is a critical nutrient for optimal health and is best obtained from sun exposure. However, in many regions, sunlight occurs for only a few months of the year. If you are fortunate enough to live in an area that receives regular sunshine, go ahead and reap its benefits often. Most of the concern about sun exposure and skin cancer is based on false alarm notions. For most people, the benefits of natural vitamin D from sunshine outweigh the slight risk of skin cancer.

Vitamins D, K1, and K2 are also present in many healthy foods. Eggs and mushrooms are both excellent sources of vitamin D. (Remember when preparing meals that vitamin D is fat-soluble, meaning it is only effective when consumed with some type of fat.) Vitamin K1 is present in dark vegetables, like kale and spinach, while vitamin K2 can be obtained from animal fats and egg yolks.

GMO, Herbicides & Pesticides

GMOs - Genetically Modified Organisms, are the result of a laboratory process where genes from the DNA of one species are extracted and artificially forced into the genes of an unrelated plant or animal. The foreign genes may come from bacteria, viruses, insects, animals or even humans.

Seeds have to be genetically modified to be able to handle the pesticides and herbicides, otherwise they would die. Instead, they can be sprayed from when they sprout until two days before they're harvested. Unfortunately, all the microorganisms in the earth are killed, and the plants don't have the nutrients they used to have.

Unfortunately, that is not the only thing happening. By eating these foods, we also become genetically modified. The extent of this vast experiment with all humans becoming guinea pigs is not known yet, but every day new diseases appear. Whether they come from the GMOs or from all the toxins is not quite clear, but the toxins from the spraying is definitely showing negative results very rapidly.

A little history:

In the late 1990s, the different GMO companies pooled money together, spending $50 million a year for five years to convince Americans and other developed country citizens that GMOs were needed to feed the world. This has become the background story, even though it's entirely untrue.

the UN and the World Bank sponsored the most comprehensive evaluation ever conducted on how to feed the world, and it was called the ISTAD report. It was written by other 400 scientists who spent years writing this report. It basically said that, "GMOs have nothing to offer to feed the hungry world, eradicate poverty, or create sustainable agriculture."

One of the co-chairman said, "It's basically a solution looking for a problem." It doesn't actually solve anything. It doesn't solve that problem. The New York Times did an analysis and found out that it didn't increase yield.

The Union of Concerned Scientists wrote a report: Failure to Yield. Where the average GMO does not increase yield and under the best scenario, it was a 0.3 percent increase per year because it was killing the corn borer in certain regions. However, agroecological solutions and organic solutions can double yield in developing countries.

People were led to believe this was for the good for many – starving people – and we in the first world countries should embrace and support it.

When we look at the future statistics, like by 2032, one in two kids will be on the autism spectrum. You look at one in three people over the age of 65 by 2050, and they will have Alzheimer's.

Roundup, sold by Monsanto, contains glyphosate, and is both a herbicide and pesticide, sprayed in the beginning only on genetically modified organisms, like corn, soy, and cotton. The GMOs were developed by Monsanto to withstand the toxins sprayed on the plants.

Plants that are being developed now are able to absorb ten times the amount or more of this poisonous chemical on the plant itself without hurting it but will kill the weeds around it.

We're getting exposed to levels of this chemical that more and more studies are showing cause cancer, tumors, and a lot of disruption in what we call the microbiome, which is now leading to conditions like Alzheimer's, Parkinson's, diabetes, and obesity.

In 2012, a study by Stephanie Seneff, senior scientist at MIT, did one of the first studies demonstrating that this glyphosate chemical actually allows the other chemicals to affect us generationally, like mercury and lead.

The number one source of lead is from our parents, bringing it full circle.

However, the third chemical affecting four generations is glyphosate and Dr. Seneff's study shows that it allows glyphosate to basically penetrate into deeper tissue like in the brain.

Glyphosate actually acts as a facilitator for these toxins to cross the blood-brain barrier and therein lies part of the problem.

We have these three chemicals coming together and crossing into the brain, which is now explaining why we're seeing so much illness, and classical medicine is not really set up to assess all this. There are a lot of people out there who are sick in this sort of vague way. They're undiagnosed.

Look at what we've inherited.

The mercury from vaccinations. Amalgam fillings. We grew up in the mercury generation.

There is a study that showed the number of fillings in a mom's mouth is proportional to how much mercury we find in a baby's brain in autopsies.

Just remember – it's not your fault! The dentists didn't even know – though they should have! Mercury is a known toxin and many dental patients got sick, but nothing was done!

I went to a dentist with not one single filling, all teeth nice and white and he opened up almost all molars and filled them with amalgam! So, my kids got their doses, too – but they were not vaccinated, so they did OK.

Glyphosate, the main toxin in Roundup, is heat fusing glycine from aldehyde and phosphorus acid. It is so toxic that it has to be stored under water. It was used to make white phosphorus, which is a chemical weapon of war.

Now that wars are more or less over – at least as they used to be – there is a war now on insects and weeds. Since nobody wants to "weed" anymore, not only the farmers, but everybody else uses Roundup to do this job. It looks like there is Roundup in every garage in America.

Since 1974, 19 billion pounds of glyphosate has been sprayed on crops, two-thirds in the last ten years, and that poundage is probably a lot more since this was written and you read it!

The sad thing is that only one-tenth of 1 percent of this spray reaches its goal – the rest, since it is water soluble, goes into the groundwater, air, and foods. We drink, breathe, and eat glyphosate every day! Isn't that scary?

Today, allergies are more common than ever! Twenty years ago, maybe one or two kids in a classroom suffered from allergies, but it was not the norm! Today, allergic attacks are often serious, causing anaphylactic attacks or serious skin eruptions, and/or heavy duty digestive reactions!

Autism is on the rise in an alarming speed – and so is Alzheimer's and other neurological disorders.

Other disorders coming from glyphosate include:

Endocrine disrupters:

- Infertility
- Cancer
- Thyroid disorders
- Hashimoto's disorder

Neurological Disorders:

- ADD/ADHD Behavioral Disorders:
- Alzheimer's
- Hodgkin's lymphoma
- Parkinson's

Depletes micronutrients:

- Iron
- Copper and zinc, so important in autism
- Magnesium
- Manganese

To eat organic food is extremely important – I think you get that now! Even if it is more expensive than the non-organic food, sickness costs the families more in the long run! It goes for the rest of the family, too! If you, the parents get sick from non-organic foods, then what happens to the rest of the family? If the breadwinner loses their job due to illness – then what?

I am sure you are aware of the diabetes pandemic, and did you know that Alzheimer's is now called type 3 diabetes?

What we eat is what we are! Just look around! We are all overweight and many are obese! The increase in body weights have changed too during the last 25 years. This was after low fat processed foods, that were full of sugars, (because otherwise it had no taste) hit the market

– and the marketing!

Sugar is addictive, more than cocaine! And it is a GMO food!

Think again about what you give your family to eat! Think twice!!! And maybe even think again!

EMFs/EMRs

We have been bombarded with toxins for the last 60 years, maybe more, but one of our biggest threats is from Electromagnetic Fields and Electromagnetic Radio waves. This is a quite new pollution, and one we cannot see.

Since cell phones and other wireless products have come on the market, cell towers are being raised all over the world, Wi-Fi is in every home, and toddlers play with phones and tablets that emit very strong electromagnetic fields. One of the results of EMFs/EMRs is that people have started to become sick without any seemingly valid ground and that's because we can't see the toxic frequencies all around us!

There are many devices you may want to keep off at night and away from bedrooms:

- Cordless phones
- Cell phones
- Wi-Fi
- TV, video games and X-box
- Baby monitors – who thought they would be harmful, but they are emitting bad electromagnetic frequencies that are harmful for young children. It's better to leave the baby's door open so you can hear them. It's good for them to get used to noise anyway!

- Laptops
- Battery back-ups
- Chargers of all kinds
- Electric clocks, at least the ones with blue light. Clocks should not be situated closer to the bed than eight feet.
- Compact fluorescent light bulbs – mercury economy. Not only do they emit EMFs, but if they break, you have to leave the house and have the Department of Health in to clean it up, or you can die! A friend of a friend of mine tried to pick up the pieces of one of those bulbs after his reading lamp fell. He ended up in the hospital for nine months! He almost didn't make it.
- Hybrid cars! We think we are taking care of the environment, but sitting in an electromagnetic box, we can get hurt ourselves in the process!

We don't know what kind of injuries we may get from all these different devices, but many of exposed children develop asthma, others get sleep disturbances and other disorders, and not many associate these "injuries" with the different fields and frequencies.

We do know that playing on a tablet or a phone, the blue light makes the brain think it is daytime, and thus, makes it more difficult to fall asleep. And everybody needs a "downtime" between working or playing on a computer and even watching TV before going to bed.

Some children, as well as adults, totally lose their energy, others get headaches or other aches and pains.

Smart meters

Smart meters that are in use today can have detrimental effect on the whole family living close to one (they often happen to be mounted just outside a bedroom). As a result, the family often has had different complaints about not feeling well.

Many European countries have recognized smart meters as a real threat and have made certain places and buildings free from Wi-Fi.

I met a man who, for a few years, was used to holding his cell phone to his ear, until he developed a tumor in the shape of a phone, just behind the ear! He did survive the operation to remove it, but who wants to go through that?

Microwave Ovens

Microwave ovens have been around for a long time, but when you cook in them, you destroy the enzymes in the food, and the body's digestive system doesn't recognize the food as nutrition, so it tries to get rid of it in one way or another because it can't absorb it! Microwaves used to be prohibited in Russia due to the EMSs that came out of them, and also because of what they did to the food.

This generation is the first to grow up with cellphones, tablets, and computers. There are Wi-Fi and computers in schools for kids from a very early age. In Israel, they started having computers and tablets already in kindergarten. Some of the parents complained because their kids got sick with headaches and no energy. I think they're still trying to change, but the government doesn't want to be behind other European countries when it comes to education.

Children are much more vulnerable to the EMFs due to their skulls not being fully developed – so their skull bones are thinner and thus more susceptible to the frequencies. Often babies are allowed to play with their parents' phones, and they are often very close to both the phones and the tablets.

ASD kids are even more susceptible to these frequencies. Some research suggests that viruses, bacteria, and fungi make these kids more toxic. This creates more problems and more difficulty in trying to detox them. One study showed that when these children were isolated from the EMFs, it was much easier to detox them from heavy metals.

There was a study done in Bavaria Valley in 2010 where they never, ever had had Wi-Fi until 60 volunteers put up the towers. At the start of the project, the volunteers' adrenaline, noradrenaline (the stress hormones), and dopamine and phentolamine (the feel-good hormones, responsible for focusing, attention and well-being) were measured. During the first six weeks, the stress hormones shot up a lot, while the other hormones tried to compensate and calm the others down, creating sleep disorders, depression, and all kinds of issues. That was just in six weeks!

Some Solutions

Here are <u>powerful but simple tips to help lower your EMF risks.</u>

There is a lot of information about shields and protections you can use, both in the home and on the body. These can either as a pendant or a bracelet.

Turn off Wi-Fi at night. The best way is to put it on a timer, from e.g. 10 p.m. to 7 a.m. This way the body can recuperate during the night without interference from Wi-Fi.

If you have a smart meter, have it changed! You might encounter trouble, but the electric company has to comply!

Don't let your kids have the strong smart phones – they have a lot of EMFs coming out of them, which are really harmful, especially for sensitive kids!

The same goes for tablets. Many non-verbal ASD children communicate through the tablets so it would be a very good idea to get a shield or protection for them. There are also protectors that can be put on the devices themselves.

Don't use microwave ovens! They destroy the food by killing all the enzymes in the food and turning it into something else. While microwaved foods are easier to prepare, they are much more difficult to digest, so it is not only the EMFs they emit – they also destroy the nutrients in the food.

At the following website, you can find things to help you manage/eliminate EMFs in your environment. Get a meter to measure the EMFs in your house in different places: where you sleep, where your computers and TVs are, where the current comes in, etc.

You know about your child's toxins. Above we talked about EMFs and frequencies, but one of the most important treatments to do is to detox. I know how difficult it is to do some of the cleansing therapies out there, especially for your child and people in the same situation. I have come across detox through ionization therapy that is mild, has no side effects, and delivers only good results. I use it myself and love the results!

Ionization Therapy for Clearing Toxins

What Is Ionization Therapy?

The IonCleanse by AMD's proprietary and patented technology results in only biocompatible electrical frequencies entering the water. Biocompatible frequencies elicit a relaxation response in the body; concurrently, they create an ionic field that cleanses and purifies the body through the healing power of ions.

The IonCleanse process ionizes the water, as H_2O is split into OH- and H+ ions. These ions attract and neutralize oppositely charged toxins. After the process, the user feels invigorated, refreshed, and relaxed.

"The IonCleanse® by AMD helps the body detox through the healing power of ions. Ions, because of their powerful charge, cleanse the body more effectively than any other method of detox. The process is safe, relaxing, and non-invasive, with no harmful side effects."

We are living in a time of the most polluted environment in earth's known history. We are continually inhaling and assimilating residues from petrochemicals, plastics, and pesticides that occupy cell receptor sites and block hormone utilization.

With the increased exposure to petrochemicals, heavy metals, and other chemicals and toxins in the environment, it is logical to assume that an ongoing detoxification program – the act of minimizing toxic accumulations in the body – will reduce the incidence of chronic degenerative diseases and improve overall quality of life.

AMD: The Foot Bath

Clearing the body of toxins is another very important step in your child's improvement health-wise!

There are many different ways to detox, but you have to be very careful in the beginning. Don't start too quickly!

You want the children to be able to feel better before you start to detox or they will feel worse, and you don't want that! You're working on making them feel happy and healthy, not sick! A heavy detox can often make them very sick! It can make anybody feel quite yucky, and I am always very careful advising use of some of the detoxes that are so popular nowadays.

There are homeopathic remedies for detox that are pretty mild and easy to dispense since they are in liquid drops. They are directed to the kidneys, colon, and liver respectively, and you can direct detoxing to one organ at a time.

If the children are very sensitive, they may not even be able to do a homeopathic remedy, and that is why I recommend an ionic foot bath. It has to be the one that detoxes with both positive and negative ions though! There are cheaper versions on the market, but they only detox single ions and are not giving the result you are looking for!

You could find a practitioner, or you can buy the machine yourself if you can afford to. I recommend you get the machine after you have tried it out. It will make it cheaper in the long run, and you can use it for the whole family. Believe me, we are all toxic!

The name of the device is AMD, which stands for "A Major Difference", which is also the name of the website. If you want to see videos about these treatments, go to You-Tube and search for AMD foot bath.

Doctor Dietrich Klinghardt, a German medical doctor, who has been working both in Washington state and in Germany with Lyme disease, autism and other ASDs and auto immune disorders for many years and with great results, uses and recommends only the AMD machine.

Debbie Floyd, mother of an autistic son and health practitioner working with autistic children, had given up on her son's possibility of becoming better. She had decided to quit all allopathic treatments and love her son just the way he was.

Another practitioner called her two days after Debbie had made her decision not to do any more treatments and asked her to try one more thing – the AMD foot bath. She agreed, and within four months her son went from starting to look into her eyes, being able to say single words, becoming potty trained and at the end of the four months saying whole sentences and having a conversation. The boy at this time was about eight years old.

This was miraculous! Debbie started to use the machine in her own office with great results. The AMD company also does research which shows improvement in these children.

The treatments can sometimes make the child have a setback, but that only shows that the treatments are working! They may seem to regress, but then they go forward. The kids, often hyperactive, are calm and still and even ask for their treatments!

It can be used for all ages. They have great results with children who are non-verbal – maybe because the change is so great and so profound, it is so noticeable!

Changes in teenagers, both developmentally and health-wise are undeniable. Teenagers, who seem untreatable, have 67 percent less of their typical symptoms after being treated with the AMD foot bath!

Other kids have 37–57 percent improvement, which is pretty remarkable, too!

The best results seem to be doing the detox three days in a row and then one day off, and then repeat. The foot bath treatments facilitate the body's release of all the toxins and gunk that it can't use.

When the person can't detox, the body can turn into channelopathy. Channelopathy can be caused by, and can create gene mutations, autoimmune disorders, and more. This means that the methylation process can't take place, the transport system doesn't work, and the poor body gets sicker and sicker.

The body then can't absorb nutrients either, which in turn means that not only can't the toxins be released, but also the nutrition uptake is blocked and therefore blocking the channels even more.

The ion detoxification when done properly, creates harmonic frequencies in the body, so a relaxation response can be reached. The goal is to activate the parasympathetic nervous system (PNS) and create rest and digestion; and stimulate the body's innate process to be able to open these blocked pathways and release everything it cannot utilize, whether it is toxins or built-up nutrition that was meant to help them, but now can't absorb it.

That's the system that we use to move these things out of the body to be able to create homeostasis.

The purpose of ion detoxification is to facilitate the body as an external proxy, where the body is compromised and can't do it on its own. This can facilitation can occur even when other internal interventions are not working.

It's quite simple when you think in terms of being able to access these frequencies that help our body come back to balance.

We're looking for grounding, for being able to create homeostasis in a way we can't do on our own anymore. It gives the body the opportunity to eliminate everything it knows is a hazard to it.

It doesn't kill the viral load, mycoplasma toxins, or other bugs. It is a supportive device that works with the body's innate system and wakes it up, so it can do what it is supposed to do.

It works together with your other protocols – diet, allergy elimination lifestyle, and other adjunctive treatments you're doing. It should always be utilized with your other practices. The only thing you can't do in conjunction is any type of other detox treatments. Those would be too harsh and dangerous.

If you have your child being treated with the ion cleanse in addition to any other protocol, the outcome can be dramatic! When the pathways are blocked and the transport system is malfunctioning, you can use any protocol all day long, but it may not go where it needs to go to be effective.

If you have a tool like the AMD ion cleanse, it can open that transport system and draw out the stuff that is backlogged so the treatments can go where they need to go, and you're going to have a profound healing experience.

The results can be remarkable. Patients who don't respond to other treatments seem to be the ones who have the best results.

Adding the AMD to your protocols could be the difference between remission or recovery

– and getting your life back!

Adenosine triphosphate (ATP) is the energy currency of life. ATP is a high -energy molecule found in every cell, and its job is to store and supply the cell with needed energy. When going through detox, any detox, you're burning ATP at much higher rate than normally. The fuel that you're burning is made of minerals. Therefore, it is important to make sure you give the person being treated, good, mineral rich food, found in dark veggies, fish, pumpkin seeds, lentils and legumes and much more.

When going through detox, any detox, the ATP (Adenosine triphosphate is the energy currency of life. ATP is a high energy molecule found in every cell, and its job is to store and supply the cell with needed energy) you're burning ATP at much higher rate than normally. The fuel that you're burning is minerals. Make sure you give the person being treated, good, mineral rich food, found in dark veggies, fish, pumpkin seeds, lentils and legumes and much more.

It is very important to keep doing the other treatments also, eliminating allergies, doing their diet and any other kind of therapy that is favorable and give results.

The ion bath is creating detoxification systemically. Once rest and digestion is activated and working inside the natural system of the body, all the organ systems in the body have the capacity of detoxification – the lung system, liver system, kidney system, and the colon will all be working on their own, doing what they are supposed to do!

If you own the system, you can help the whole family to detox since we're all toxic! Think about it: babies are born with close to 200 different toxins in their umbilical cord – that's what the mother transfers to the child! So, everybody would do very well using the ionic foot bath. Just don't settle for the inexpensive one from somewhere online! Make sure you know what you are buying. It has to work with both the negative and positive ions!

This system was not created for autism specifically. It was and is used for MS, Arthritis, Alzheimer's, etc. with good results, where there were none before. So, this is another reason to treat the whole family!

conclusion

I have talked about different ways and possibilities in changing your child's and your family's lives through using food as medicine, eliminating allergies, changing lifestyle, and detoxification.

I have shown you different diets that will help your child with their well-being, reactions, and symptoms. I have talked about vaccinations and their pitfalls, and the importance of eating organic, non-GMO foods.

I hope you now can see, that there are many things that can be done to make your child's life better and that it is possible to have a happy, healthy family by changing lifestyle and eliminating allergies. The whole family will feel and act better, and you may see progress in as little as a couple of weeks.

There are other resources, too! Suzy Miller, who used to be a speech therapist for autistic kids, had an experience one day when she saw her little patient, four years old, who was totally non-verbal, coming up to her. She heard in her head that he saluted her with: *Hello Master*!

First, she didn't know what to think – she was not into telepathy or ESP, or anything like that. But what she found was the start of another way to communicate with these children. She now has courses for parents where they learn how to communicate with their kids! She calls it Awesomism and has a book on Amazon called the same.

Another relatively new treatment is with stem cells. The recommended treatment center is in Mexico, highly up-to-date, and meets the FDA's strict cGTP guidelines.

I have a dream that kids with ASD can eat foods that are healthy, GMO and herbicide/pesticide free.

I have a dream that they can eat and be in environments that don't make them have temper tantrums, because they have an allergic reaction to something that makes them feel horrible and nobody knows why they're behaving badly.

I have a dream that parents will be able to decide for themselves, when and if to expose their children to vaccinations, after the doctors give them an honest answer to the risks. Make the doctors explain that a child's brain barrier is not developed until they're about three years of age and before that, all the neurotoxins in the vaccines go directly to their young brains.

I have a dream that although there may always be autism or other neurological disorders, these people and kids are healthy and happy.

For this to happen, parents need to be informed and this is my mission – to inform you about possibilities of being healthy, eating healthy – knowing what food is good to eat and what is not; knowing where to buy your food; teaching you how to eliminate allergies and how to live in a clean, non-toxic environment.

Are you ready to start a movement for healthy, happy kids and families?

Testimonials

From Christine, mother of three

"I had been suffering from severe allergies for ten years. I have three children, a ten -year-old boy, an eight-year-old girl, and an eight-month-old baby also with allergies. When I was pregnant the last time, all my symptoms and allergies got worse. My baby daughter soon developed an allergy to dairy and gluten that I found out through testing and was losing weight slowly, so between her and the behavioral problems with my son, that I didn't even know had to do with allergies, and my own allergies, I was at my wits' end and purchased The Allergy Kit. I was tired of just treating the symptoms, I had been around the block so many times; I was desperately looking for a solution. I was looking everywhere and finally found The Allergy Kit and felt at peace. I knew I had found the help I was looking for.

How it would help and how quickly it would help – I was floored by – to be honest, I had suffered so long, that I thought it would take a miracle.

Nourishing my third child, being so sick, I was just wiped, extreme fatigue, hard to breathe and my asthma – all my symptoms were just magnified. I was dragging through each day and with three children it is very difficult; I was des-

perate to find something. So, symptoms – hard to breathe, a very, very chronic runny nose. I have this progressive twitch, interrupting my sleep at night and severe vertigo, which is very scary. If I get an attack and the children are not here and with the baby, who is going to help me?

And this quality of life – sleeping, always feeling too cold, lots of neurological symptoms, difficulty thinking and focusing, and I have suffered from depression from my second child, very severe for ten to twelve months. I've just had struggles with a lot of allergies and taken tons of medications – you can say I have tried it all, I have been around the block – I'm done!

When I started the kit, the very first thing I noticed was with my son. It was amazing, after the very first vial, after 48 hours, he was a completely different child. We had moved from up north to Colorado, and two years later we noticed that his nose was running and didn't make the connection to food allergies. We thought it was environmental, so we didn't realize the severe egg allergy he had, so two days after, we could not ever get him, for the last 9 months, to sit down at the dinner table with us. We had tried everything, it didn't matter what we did or didn't do, he would not sit down with us and we really thought it was a behavior issue. He was very aggressive with his sister, very short tempered with her. He hadn't played with her for the last 9 months, and that was gone in 48 hours!

He was a completely 360 degrees different child! He sat at the dinner table! After the fifth night of sitting at the dinner table, I said to my husband, "Can you believe this?

He has sat down at the dinner table the whole week and we hadn't said a word to him. To sit down, don't touch that or don't do that. We sat down and had a peaceful dinner!" His sister would play with him again and was having a good time again. You know, before I had to tend to her and tend to him and to the baby. They were like three separate beings, they couldn't do anything together, because of his issues, so it really restored the peace in the family. There are so many things, we can't put words to that, just that the quality of life with your family, that when it was gone and you don't realize how much you miss that. I can hardly talk about it without crying!

That was the very first thing that we really noticed. My oldest daughter, she had a dairy allergy, a severe form with hives and eczema, so I started to give her medication, so she wouldn't get scarring, not too long ago, and then, again. The first week after the first vial, we stopped giving her the medication to see how the dairy was doing on her, and – nothing! No tearing of the skin on the back of her legs, no itchy bumps, no welts, no nothing, so I asked her if she was sure she ate dairy that day? And she said, "Yes, mom, I had the same cheese, I had the same milk, I had the same thing, nothing different!"

You get scared and think surely, it's going to reappear, and it doesn't, you can't believe your eyes, it's crazy!

My youngest daughter, after the fifth vial, her bowel movements are back to normal, which they have not been since I started to give her solid food. They had been horrible, so her weight gain has been very slow, due to her poor nutrition, her ability to absorb the food because of her intestinal allergy. It's great to see the change in her abdomen and her hair is growing!

The crazy thing is we haven't finished the kit yet! We still have the grains to do and the environmentals! I am so excited! What more is to come? We're not even done! It has already helped the environmental allergies! With all the tree pollen here right now, and my nose hardly drips at all!

Before I would live with paper tissues stuffed in my nose when sleeping. My nose would be torn, and I couldn't leave my house; it was terrible!

So annoying and now – nothing! That's why I have a bag of hope, especially with myself. I had given up on hope. I looked at this as "this is what I am looking forward to for the rest of my life," to have these kinds of symptoms and lack of quality of life. And you know, you can't see it as with a broken arm or a broken leg. People can't see inside your head, how you feel, but when you're suffering like that and you're treating symptoms with drugs that don't help you feel any better, they don't do anything. It gets hard to get up. I want to raise these three children. Now I can do that! I am so happy – I couldn't be happier, truly!"

Lucy and Jack

I had a patient, Lucy, who I had treated for an illness nobody could "fix," and she herself said it started after a spider bite. I treated her with the kit and for the spider bite and she totally recuperated!

She had a grandson, who had been diagnosed with autism and recommended that her daughter see me. He used to have at least seven temper tantrums per day and they couldn't take him along to places he didn't know because if they did, he would have a meltdown.

He only wanted to wear certain clothes and shoes. Food was another problem; he craved sugars and sugary foods and would scream until the mother broke down and gave him what he wanted. His digestive system was not very good either and that was probably the reason for his out-breaks– he was in pain!

At the first consultation, she brought along Jack, who was quite "lively," interrupted the whole time and ran around. He didn't make eye contact and his speech was very limited. When he got too excited, the mother pulled out a two-foot-long gummy snake, and while I gasped, he started to eat it! He was quiet as long as he was eating, which was the mother's idea, but then he got the sugar high! It was not better.

I started his treatments. Some days he would come in with a thread around his finger, totally absorbed in the thread, not aware of his surroundings. Other days he was just wild and we had to use a surrogate and one more person to treat him!

After the third treatment his speech started to improve considerably. As a matter of fact, the family took him out of his speech therapy!

He started to have eye contact with people, even the ones he didn't know! The improvement was miraculous!

I didn't see him after the first ten treatments - they found another practitioner closer to home.

One day the father came for a treatment and I asked him about Jack. The answer was that he was totally normal, going to normal school, and reading on one level higher than his class. The dad was very proud of him.

The grandmother called me several times thanking me for saving her grandson's life!

I saw Jack again ten years later. He had some anger issues due to some allergies coming back because his diet was horrible! He only needed a couple of treatments this time and then he was good to go!

I don't think the mother changed his diet too much! I don't think she really believed in it, but he became a totally healthy child anyway, just from eliminating the allergies! Not changing the diet is not the norm, because as you can see, it is a very important part for the journey to recuperation!

Michael

Michael, an 11-year-old boy, very big for his age, was brought in by his mother, who was my patient.

She was a school teacher and her son was in special education class due to his bad behavior, and because he was thought of to be "slow."

The mother was very intimidated by her son being in special ed class and was also very upset with his behavior, not only in school. He was disrespectful to her and to his grandparents, too. There was constant fighting.

After a few treatments, his behavior changed completely. One day after coming home from grocery shopping, the mom went to the bathroom and when she came out, he had put away the groceries and was on his way to throw away the garbage! This was a first! It had never happened before, and from that day on, he changed so much he was moved from the special ed. class, and went on to become an honor student until he graduated high school! I lost contact with him after they moved, but I will never forget him and his fabulous results.

Grace

Little Grace, a beautiful girl, 3 years old, suffered from bad rashes and eczema that was very itchy. After the first treatment, her eczema got better – she had been allergic to chicken and that was what the mother would give her almost every day!

Most of the time we don't think about these reactions and where they come from!

Acknowledgments

In writing this book I have been helped by my angels from weekly meetings in Jean Slatter's Creative Mystic Group, where I was picked up if I thought it was too difficult or I couldn't do it. Donna and Mary Ellen helped me with the editing.

I am grateful to Angela Lauria, who gave me inspiration and ideas I hadn't thought about myself, that changed my way of doing things!

About the Author

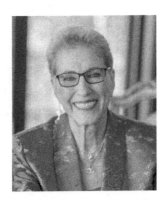

Ynge Ljung, acupuncture physician, naturopath and the creator of The Allergy Kit, graduated from the Community School of Traditional Chinese Medicine in 1995.

Taking many courses in additional modalities, she studied the NAET system for allergy elimination in 1998 and added this modality to her acupuncture practice. She had found, that acupuncture being a great medicine, wasn't always enough and adding allergy elimination to her treatments enhanced the results.

The trend today to be gluten sensitive, for example, has become a pandemic, and so have allergies in general.

Digestion is getting worse, people and children are getting sicker every day, bad health has become not only an epidemic, but a pandemic, which means health is declining all over the world.

This has been of great concern to Ynge, who during these last 20 years has seen the health decline also in children. One in two children has chronic illness, and one child in twenty-five runs the risk of becoming autistic!

Why? That's the question she is trying to answer, or at least to inform the mothers, fathers, and caregivers of these sick children.

She is passionate about better knowledge of nutrition, vaccinations, what our crops are sprayed with, genetically modified organisms, what all these things can possibly do to our health, and why it is so important to eat organic food so that we can improve our health and our children's future. Ynge has a clinic in Hallandale, Florida and she is also available for remote consultations.

Thank You

Thank you for reading to the end of this book and joining the journey to find your lost child!

Please visit the Website: www.TheAllergyKit.com

To further connect with Ynge Ljung and access bonus content:

- Recommended Reading
- Instructions for Muscle Testing
- Additional Resources
- And More!

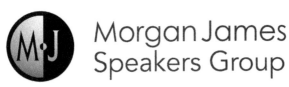

Morgan James
Speakers Group

www.TheMorganJamesSpeakersGroup.com

We connect Morgan James published
authors with live and online events
and audiences who will benefit
from their expertise.

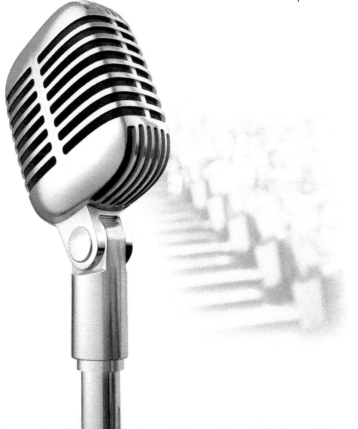

Morgan James makes all of our titles available
through the Library for All Charity Organization.

www.LibraryForAll.org